THE EXERCISE FACTOR

"Jim Kirwan gets the most important thing exactly right: exercise is the heart (and maybe the soul) of the good life. You may love it, you may hate it... doesn't matter. If you have a sane bone in your body you will put exercise at or very near the center of your life... and one of your most basic commitments. Read Jim's book, do the exercise... live the great life."

—**Chris Crowley** Best Selling Author, *Younger Next Year*

"With so many fitness and exercise books on the market it is hard to know which ones to buy. Jim Kirwan's *The eXercise Factor* is a must for your fitness library. He is such a motivator and his book is easy to read and even easier to follow. Jim has a fail-proof formula that makes sense and results in moving more, having more energy, and making changes that will change your life!"

—**Janis Newton** Program Director Healthy Charleston Challenge, Interim Director MUSC Wellness Center

"Lots of straight talk and common sense motivation about the value of exercise. Jim Kirwan challenges every reader to alter our thoughts and actions about sensible exercise, good nutrition and enhancement of the quality of life. He blows a hole in traditional excuses for not exercising."

—**William R. Barfield, Ph.D., FACSM**, Professor, Health and Human Performance, College of Charleston, Adjunct Professor, Department of Orthopaedics, MUSC

"This book is so true to life and the benefits of keeping your body moving. Jim Kirwan's passion for sports and inspiring people to get involved in activities is like a Domino Effect! Pass it on!"

—**Julian Smith** Race Director, Cooper River Bridge Run

"When it comes to exercise, Jim Kirwan knows what's up. His simple approach to exercise will elevate everything in your life, and is essential for health, happiness, and a long high quality life! He has your back!"

—**Carrie Roldan** The Run Yourself Happy Coach

"Sedentary activity and lack of discipline in life choices may accelerate the aging process, often with irreversible physical consequences. Jim Kirwan succeeds in communicating the lifelong merits of exercise for all, with practical guidelines to maximize wellness."

—**Dr. John M. Graham Jr., MD** Orthopaedic Surgeon,
Orthopaedic Specialists of Charleston

"Jim Kirwan is very passionate about exercise and getting people to live a healthy lifestyle. He loves teaching and he practices everything he preaches in his book *The eXercise Factor*. Jim is a visionary and sees the big picture; he sees the health and fitness needs out there and where America needs to be 10 years from now."

—**Tami Dennis** Head Coach, Mt. Pleasant Track and Field

"I see the effects of inactivity in my practice every day! With this concise and clearly written book, Jim Kirwan contrasts the increasing costs of inactivity with the many benefits of exercise. He sets out a very realistic, step-by-step approach to getting back into shape, regardless of your age, weight or current fitness level. He also challenges you to learn more about your health and diet as well as exercise and to take the necessary actions which will ultimately lead to a longer, higher quality life."

—**Thomas Keane, MD** Charleston SC

"One of the most significant factors to being unhealthy is a lack of exercise. In *The eXercise Factor* Jim tackles our population of people that are most susceptible to the pitfalls of not being active and exercising. In a safe and leveled progression of exercise, his book will ultimately lead to healthier and happier individuals."

—**Mark Rutledge PT, OCS, MHS, MTC**
President Rehabilitation Centers of Charleston

"Jim Kirwan is on a mission to get even the most inactive, out of shape adult to start to add exercise to his or her life, in order to extend and, more importantly, improve that life. In this book he proves himself a potent "eXercist", using his persuasive chants and mnemonic incantations to cast out the devils of sedentary habits and defeatist attitudes. He lays out very clearly and convincingly the reasons why everyone should exercise, and provides concrete ways to start down that more healthful road. For the person thinking about exercise but in need of encouragement and a doable starting plan, this is a great book."

—**Patrick M. O'Neil, Ph.D.** Director Weight Management Center,
Professor, Department of Psychiatry and Behavioral Sciences,
Professor, Department of Surgery, Medical University of South Carolina.

"There are many health and fitness books to choose from but none address the critical importance of exercise like *The eXercise Factor*. Yet, it is not just about exercise; there are four key drivers which work together to turbo charge your chances of living a long, high quality life: exercise, nutrition, knowledge and what Jim calls the 'X Factor'. *The eXercise Factor* will challenge you to take a long hard look at yourself. It is packed with tons of great advice and an easy-to-follow roadmap to the good life!"

—**David L. Hancock** Founder, Morgan James Publishing

THE EXERCISE FACTOR

Ease Into the Best
Shape of Your Life
Regardless of Your
Age, Weight or
Current Fitness Level

JIM KIRWAN

NEW YORK

THE EXERCISE FACTOR
Ease Into the Best Shape of Your Life Regardless of Your Age, Weight or Current Fitness Level

© 2015 **JIM KIRWAN**.

Published in New York, New York, by Morgan James Publishing. Morgan James and The Entrepreneurial Publisher are trademarks of Morgan James, LLC.
www.MorganJamesPublishing.com

The Morgan James Speakers Group can bring authors to your live event. For more information or to book an event visit The Morgan James Speakers Group at
www.TheMorganJamesSpeakersGroup.com.

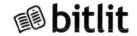

A **free** eBook edition is available
with the purchase of this print book.

CLEARLY PRINT YOUR NAME ABOVE IN UPPER CASE

Instructions to claim your free eBook edition:
1. Download the BitLit app for Android or iOS
2. Write your name in **UPPER CASE** on the line
3. Use the BitLit app to submit a photo
4. Download your eBook to any device

ISBN 978-1-63047-322-8 paperback
ISBN 978-1-63047-323-5 eBook
ISBN 978-1-63047-324-2 hardcover
Library of Congress Control Number:
2014942823

Cover Design by:
Chris Treccani
www.3dogdesign.net

Interior Design by:
Bonnie Bushman
bonnie@caboodlegraphics.com

In an effort to support local communities, raise awareness and funds, Morgan James Publishing donates a percentage of all book sales for the life of each book to Habitat for Humanity Peninsula and Greater Williamsburg.

Get involved today, visit
www.MorganJamesBuilds.com

Habitat
for Humanity®
Peninsula and
Greater Williamsburg
Building Partner

To My Dad:

His untimely passing came at a time when we were becoming good friends and it had a profound influence on my life. Who knows where I would be today; would I even be alive? I think it is safe to say I would never have written this book.

To My Mum:

I cannot dedicate this book to my dad without including my mum, because they were partners. Mum suffered more than anyone because she had to endure nearly twenty years without him.

Contents

Acknowledgments   xi

Introduction   xiii

Part 1: You Can Choose To Bypass Normal Aging   **1**

            Introduction To Part 1   3

Chapter 1   Why Is Exercise So Important?   5

Chapter 2   The Vast Majority Of Americans Do Not Exercise Enough   14

Chapter 3   Major Causes Of The Inactivity Epidemic   24

Chapter 4   What Are You Going To Do?   36

Chapter 5   Your Four Key Drivers Of Success   44

Part 2: Exercise—The Secret Sauce To A Great Life   **47**

            Introduction To Part 2   49

Chapter 6   Thirteen Obstacles To Exercise   51

Chapter 7   How To Make Exercise A High Priority In Your Life   62

Chapter 8   How Long Should You Spend Exercising?   72

Chapter 9   What Type Of Exercise Should You Do?   85

Chapter 10   How To Allocate Your Exercise Time   104

Part 3: Turbocharge Your Life With The X Factor   **115**

              Introduction To Part 3   117

Chapter 11   The X Factor Revealed   119

Chapter 12   Your X Factor Decision   133

Chapter 13   Your Current Fitness Level   139

Chapter 14   Your Project Plan   149

Chapter 15   Your Project Implementation   160

Chapter 16   Your Project Review   173

Part 4: A Fountain Of Knowledge For Your New Lifestyle   **181**

              Introduction To Part 4   183

Chapter 17   Knowledge—Your Third Key Driver   185

Chapter 18   Mind Your Brain   195

Chapter 19   Nutrition—Your Fourth Key Driver   205

Chapter 20   How To Start Exercise In 5 Easy Steps   217

Chapter 21   Anyone Can Run   224

              Resources   235

              Index   238

              About The Author   241

ACKNOWLEDGMENTS

There are a few people who influenced my decision to write this book and I want to acknowledge their help and support.

I attended Brendon Burchard's 10X Publishing conference in December 2012 and left after three days inspired by Brendon to write a book. Nine months later he referred my proposals for *The eXercise Factor* to publishers Morgan James. Special thanks to their founder, David Hancock and his team for their encouragement and support throughout the project.

To Lianne Sánchez who edited my manuscript and to the following who endorsed my book:

Bill Barfield

Chris Crowley

Tami Dennis

John Graham

David Hancock

Tom Keane

Janis Newton

Pat O'Neil

Carrie Roldan

Mark Rutledge

Julian Smith

Special thanks to Janis Newton, the Interim Director of the MUSC Wellness Center and Program Director of the Healthy Charleston Challenge. Letting me speak to the participants of the Challenge over the last six or seven years has changed the course of my life and was a big factor in the creation of Get America Moving and writing my book.

To my daughter Meghan and my son James, who, I am proud to say, totally buy into and are great examples of how to live a healthy and high quality life. Last but definitely not least, I cannot ever thank my wife Maureen enough for her support, love and especially her patience with me during this project.

INTRODUCTION

Despite all the benefits of exercise and the juicy carrot of a longer, higher quality life, the vast majority of Americans do not exercise enough.

I came to America back in 2003 to set up a new retail business called TrySports in Mt. Pleasant, South Carolina and I was on a mission to encourage people to try the aerobic activities of walking, running, swimming, cycling and fitness in general. I love living here in America and have witnessed many positive developments. However, when it comes to our health problems, very little has changed and obesity, diabetes and Alzheimer's are at epidemic proportions. Underlying these three major health concerns is what I call the Inactivity Epidemic and because of it, I stepped down from my position as CEO of TrySports and I am now on a mission to Get America Moving!

This is my fourth major career change and they always remind me of one of my favorite songs, *"I still haven't found what I'm looking for"* from U2, my favorite band. At last, I think I have found what I am looking for!

From the moment we are born to the day we die, exercise is beneficial, yet clearly there are many obstacles which stop us in our tracks, especially as we get older. But it doesn't matter if you are young or old, normal weight, overweight or obese, active or sedentary, exercise will help you.

Growing Up

Exercise is in our DNA and once babies learn to walk it is hard to stop them. Of course, we don't describe what they are doing as exercise but it is, and they are having great fun doing it. Likewise, as babies grow into kids they continue to play; exercise is a fundamental part of everything they do, though unfortunately this is changing.

When I was a kid growing up in Ireland back in the sixties, we used to "go out to play" and all we did was play games which involved running, chasing, climbing, jumping and dancing. Our parents didn't have to check to see if we were getting the minimum recommended daily amount of exercise (one hour) because unless we were sick, we far exceeded the minimum every day and largely because of that, only a very small minority of kids were overweight.

As we moved into our teens the games we played turned into impromptu soccer and tip-rugby matches and we never got bored with them. This physical activity is what I refer to as unplanned exercise and was in addition to all the planned exercise we did growing up, which in my case included Gaelic football and hurling, soccer, swimming, a little cricket and a lot of rugby.

Kids today seem to grow up much faster and their interests are different. While they continue to play planned sports, I fear that much of the unplanned activities that I did have been replaced with more sedentary pursuits which focus on their iPhones, iPads, Xboxes and other computer games. With all the technological "progress" during this time I believe we have unwittingly made a serious mistake that we need to rectify quickly.

Our Adult Years

Why do so many adults retire from exercise in their early- to mid-thirties?

As kids grow into adults, many play their favorite sports at college and beyond. However, slowly but surely, family and work responsibilities begin to take over. Around the same time they find it increasingly difficult to keep up with their much younger teammates and competitors and so one by one they retire with very few lasting into their late thirties. Now this is perfectly understandable, but should they retire from exercise altogether?

This is an important question which I feel very strongly about because my dad stopped exercising in his early thirties and this was a major factor in his premature death some fifteen years later at the far too early age of forty-seven.

My Dad

I had just celebrated my twentieth birthday a week earlier, with hardly a care in the world. My dad's death was a huge shock at the time and I never saw it coming. I had just come home from a Friday night out with some pals, at about midnight. On my way to and from the bathroom, I saw him in his bedroom with his back to the door and I never said good night! When I got up on Saturday morning, my sister told me that he wasn't feeling well and that mum had brought him to St. Vincent's, the local hospital. He died early that morning of a massive heart attack in the ER.

I will always remember my mum's face through the front window as she walked to the hall door; I knew before she said anything that Dad was not coming home. I knew he was on medication for angina, which in hindsight obviously didn't work very well. He didn't smoke or drink but was probably about ten or fifteen pounds overweight and I also think he was under some stress at work. The one thing I know for sure, however, is that, like nearly all his contemporaries, he didn't exercise. He "retired" from playing rugby around thirty-two years of age and for the next fifteen years, except for the occasional walk and the very odd game of golf, dad didn't exercise.

Unfortunately, we knew very little about the benefits of exercise and good nutrition back in the mid-seventies; while we know a lot more now, you would not think so based on the lifestyle of the average person. That moment I saw my dad for the last time is frozen in my memory as if it happened yesterday. He would be eighty-six today if he was alive; that's thirty-nine lost years. I don't want what happened to him and to me to happen to you or your kids.

While we cannot control the future and there are no guarantees, I believe there is much we can do. There is no reason to stop exercising; sure, you might have to change your activities and slow down a bit, but stop altogether? If you stop in your mid-thirties, it is hardly a surprise that you don't exercise as you get older. But here's the thing—the less exercise you do, the earlier you will start aging. Surely it would be better to postpone the aging process for as long as you can. The good news is you can do that with exercise and it is never too late to start!

Overweight

If you need to lose weight, the sooner you start exercising and the more you do, the quicker you will lose the weight. Yes, it will be tough but you can do it and you will get there if you put your heart and soul into it.

I'm sure you're familiar with the television show *The Biggest Loser*. Think about the competitors at the start of the competition; they are motivated but apprehensive and they are right to be because it turns out to be a real struggle. But they persevere and a few short months later they are transformed. Now "in real life" it will typically take longer but the principles remain the same! The combination of exercise and a healthy diet of good food will turbo charge your efforts to lose weight. While losing weight is important, there are even greater prizes to be won, including an increase in your life expectancy and an improved quality of life.

Inactive

If you are currently inactive or just dabble with exercise, it is never too late to start all over again. Of course, you need to proceed with caution and go slowly, moving forward gradually, step by step, day by day, week by week. This will be tough and it will require commitment and resilience but you can make it to the Promised Land. Many have made it before you and many will after you; if you believe in yourself, you will, too!

Exercise is a critical part of the solution to our health problems in America and all across the world. The evidence is overwhelming that physical activity helps you increase your life expectancy and with it, perhaps more importantly, the quality of your life. I feel so strongly about this that I have created my own health and fitness motto so that I can continuously reinforce the point. So here it is:

"You don't have to be Fit and Healthy to Start
but you do have to Start to be Fit and Healthy!"

The word "start" is self-explanatory but I use it as an easy-to-remember acronym, which I discuss in detail in Chapter 20: How to Start Exercise in 5 Easy Steps. You can also find a few television interviews on this topic on the Get America Moving website in the blog and media areas (**www.GetAmericaMoving.com**).

So whether you are doing too little or no exercise at all, there is no better time than the present to get started.

My Objective For This Book

About seven years ago, I was invited to speak at the Healthy Charleston Challenge, which is sometimes described as our local version of *The Biggest Loser* television show. It's run by the MUSC (Medical University of South Carolina) Wellness Department and it is essentially a chronic disease prevention program that deals with overweight and obesity and helps change the way participants live their lives.

I present twice each year and while my presentation continues to evolve, my objective for the participants has essentially remained the same:

> *To reinforce the Challenge objectives and inspire the participants to continue their new journey no matter what, and to focus on the key drivers of their new lifestyle, including nutrition and especially exercise.*

You may or may not see yourself as a *Healthy Charleston Challenge* or *Biggest Loser* candidate because, unlike the participants, maybe you haven't started your new lifestyle yet or maybe you are not overweight. But if you are reading this book you are probably concerned about one or more aspects of your health, such as your weight and fitness, and you have decided you want to do something about it.

Maybe your concern is for a family member or friend or maybe you just want to learn more and continue to improve your health. Whatever the reason, my objective for you is largely the same. Like the Challenge participants, I hope to persuade and inspire you to start or continue your new lifestyle and to focus on my *Four Key Drivers of Success,* outlined in Chapter 5.

In Part 1, I will show you how to bypass normal aging and increase your life expectancy and especially the quality of your life. In Part 2, our focus is exercise, the secret sauce to a great life and I will explain why it must be a high priority in your life. In Part 3, I will show you how to turbo charge your exercise and your life with the X Factor and finally, in Part 4, we will discuss the importance of knowledge, especially relating to your health and nutrition in your new lifestyle.

Medical Clearance

You should always visit your doctor before you start a new exercise program, including any of the ideas presented in this book. It is always better to have your doctor's support and guidance, as he or she is familiar with your unique set of circumstances. Armed with their support and encouragement, you are all set to start your new journey!

PART I

YOU CAN CHOOSE TO
BYPASS NORMAL AGING

INTRODUCTION TO PART 1

In Part 1 of *The eXercise Factor*, my primary goal is to show you that you can choose to bypass normal aging. However, knowing that you can and wanting to are not quite the same so I also have to persuade you that by choosing to bypass normal aging, you will make a great decision, not just for you but for your family and friends.

In **Chapter 1**, I explain why exercise is so important to your health and to a high quality life. We know that exercise is good for us and has many health benefits, yet I believe the vast majority of Americans do not exercise enough. I address three major health problems: obesity, diabetes and Alzheimer's and I introduce you to the silent killer which I call the Inactivity Epidemic.

In **Chapter 2**, I seek to validate my hypothesis that the vast majority of Americans do not exercise enough. To help me do this, I refer to three important sources of information: the official American view, which is reinforced by the rest of the world view and some great news from a major research study.

In **Chapter 3**, I explain how we have arrived at this point. There are many reasons why this has happened and we will review some of the major causes of the Inactivity Epidemic. However, I believe that ultimately you will have to take control of your own destiny. You have a choice; you can make either good decisions or bad ones. No one else can do this for you.

In **Chapter 4**, I ask you a very simple but serious question – what are you going to do? To help you make the right decision, I explain life expectancy from both a quantitative and qualitative perspective. We also consider if life expectancy is just a throw of the dice and finally I show you that you can choose to bypass normal aging but you have to make the decision and then do it.

In **Chapter 5**, the final chapter of Part 1, I introduce you to the four key drivers of success, which are discussed in the rest of the book.

CHAPTER 1

WHY IS EXERCISE SO IMPORTANT?

We all know that vegetables are good for us, but just because they are doesn't mean we will eat them. In a similar way we all know that exercise is good for us and has many health benefits, but for the vast majority of Americans, it suffers the very same fate as the vegetables.

Some of us have learned that we can enhance the spinach or kale and this turns it from boring and distasteful into a much more satisfying and enjoyable experience. Likewise with exercise, some of us have learned that exercise is not just enjoyable and great fun—it can even be addictive. To simplify this, let's say there are just two groups of people: the small minority who love exercise and probably do more than enough, and the vast majority who don't exercise enough. The challenge we face, and it is a very substantial one, is to find ways to get increasing numbers to convert from the majority to the minority, so that in time the minority can become the majority.

Why are exercise lovers such a small minority? How have we arrived at this point? Why do so many Americans love sports and yet see exercise as a waste of their time? Or if they do exercise, why is it often seen as a chore they want to get out of the way as quickly as possible?

My Journey to the USA

Initially when I came to the USA in 2003, I was on a mission to set up a new business in the triathlon field. When I was younger I played many different sports, though rugby was always my first choice. As I moved into my late twenties, I knew I could not continue playing rugby forever so I decided to transition to running to stay in good shape. As time passed, it became my new first choice of exercise, though rugby is still the sport I love the most. As my passion for running intensified, I completed a few marathons during the eighties, but unfortunately for me they took their toll on my body, especially on my lower back. This was a weak spot after a few injuries I had gotten while playing rugby.

In the nineties, triathlons became my passion. What I love about the sport of triathlon is the variety of activity—swimming, cycling and running. While it is definitely a challenge, it is a realistic one. Best of all, unlike many other "adult" sports, such as tennis or golf, no specialized talent is required (although, of course, you do have to be able to swim, bike and run). Hard work and the will to succeed are necessary, but thankfully for me these were not an issue.

After researching triathlon business opportunities, I decided to set up a retail store in Mount Pleasant, SC. Mount Pleasant is a beautiful town with a population of 72,000 just north of Downtown Charleston, across the Cooper River. I was definitely on a mission to convert people to the sport of triathlon but I recognized quite early on that by itself it was not a viable business.

I set up TrySports in November of 2003 and we opened for business in February 2004 with the emphasis on encouraging the folks of Mount Pleasant and Charleston to "Try" the aerobic activities of walking, running, cycling, swimming and fitness, as well as triathlon.

Healthy Charleston Challenge

At TrySports, we played a proactive role in the fitness and health of our communities from the very beginning. We got involved in many local events and one of those was the Healthy Charleston Challenge. This event is organized twice yearly by the Wellness Center at the Medical University of South Carolina (MUSC), and is often described as Charleston's version of the popular "Biggest Loser" television show.

My involvement as a speaker there had a profound influence on my future, as you will discover throughout this book. At the Wellness Center, they create programs that help change the way people live their lives and the Challenge is a chronic disease prevention program that deals with overweight and obesity. My involvement with the Challenge really opened my eyes from three different perspectives.

First— that we have some major health problems in America.
Second— that we can actually do something about them and
Third— that we are not doing enough to resolve some of these major health problems.

Health of the Nation

My concern for the "Health of the Nation" has grown exponentially during the eleven years I have been living in the USA to the point that today I believe we have some critically serious health problems. What makes the situation even worse is that the problem continues to deteriorate because we are not taking it seriously enough.

I believe there is much we can do to solve the problem. I decided to call this section the "Health of the Nation" because I started writing it around the time of the annual State of the Union address by the president. As in all previous years, since I came to the USA, the address covered all the usual territory from the debt ceiling to terrorism to healthcare. But, in referring to healthcare, it failed to mention some of the greatest threats of all. For me these are not party political issues. However, since I have come to the USA, I don't think the address has ever mentioned these issues.

So I am going to address three major health problems (well four, actually) which are rightly referred to as **EPIDEMICS!** These epidemics refer to the United States but in truth, we have a world-wide pandemic.

Epidemic No. 1: Obesity

According to the Centers for Disease Control and Prevention (CDC[1]), data from the National Health and Nutrition Examination Survey 2009–2010 shows that some 36%, or more than one-third of adults aged twenty and over, are obese. Obesity prevalence did not differ much between men and women, but adults aged sixty and over were more likely to be obese than younger adults.

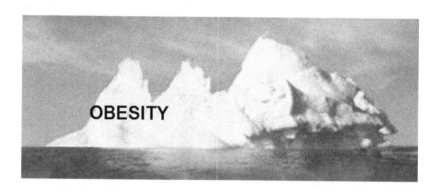

Some 17% of young people under twenty are also obese but of even greater significance is that this is triple the rate of just one generation ago. When I look back to when I went to school in the sixties and early seventies, you could count the number of overweight kids, never mind obese, on one hand. At most, one guy in my class of about a hundred males would have been considered overweight but even he was very active and played rugby; in fact, he was one of the best players in my school. It is interesting how times have changed but as I was growing up, an overweight person had some kind of health problem that was outside of his control; no one would consciously choose to be overweight, let alone obese.

Like all statistical information, the figures to which I refer above are out of date by the time they get to the people. It begs the question—has the situation gotten better or worse? Unfortunately, I believe the answer is almost certainly a negative one.

While obesity is very serious, we should be just as concerned about overweight trends.

---

1   CDC referred to NCHS Data Brief No. 82 (January, 2012)

Some 70% of Americans are now considered either overweight or obese. To me, this is an astonishing statistic and like all the others, it is trending the wrong way. You do not need to be a rocket scientist to figure out what will happen as the American population ages.

Definition of Overweight and Obese

Overweight and obese are labels for the ranges of weight that are greater than what is generally considered healthy for a given height. The terms also identify ranges of weight that have been shown to increase the likelihood of certain diseases and other health problems. For adults, overweight and obese ranges are determined by using weight and height to calculate a number call the "Body Mass Index" or BMI for short. BMI is used because for most people, it correlates with their amount of body fat.

An adult who has a BMI between 25 and 29.9 is considered overweight.

An adult who has a BMI of 30 or higher is considered obese.

Warning: While BMI provides an easy way to measure overweight and obesity, many question its accuracy and usefulness, so it should only be used as a guide.

Epidemic No. 2: Type 2 Diabetes

Type 2 diabetes is closely linked to overweight and obesity. This country has seen the number of people diagnosed with diabetes rise from 1.5 million in 1958 to 18.8 million in 2010. You can measure that increase whatever way you want, 12.5 times or 1253%, but one way or another it is an increase of epidemic proportions.

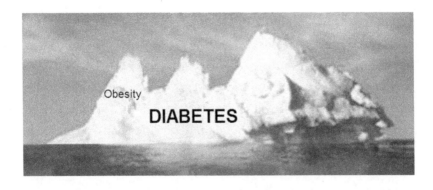

Today the National Diabetes Education Program reports that some twenty-six million Americans have diabetes. What is especially scary is that some seven million of these do not know they have the disease. Perhaps even more alarming is that it is estimated that eighty million adults aged twenty and older are considered pre-diabetic. Pre-diabetes is a condition where blood glucose levels are higher than normal but not yet high enough to be called diabetic.

One of my favorite authors is health expert Mark Hyman[2], who refers to the "Diabesity Epidemic" which combines both the obesity and diabetes epidemics into one term. It is a more comprehensive way to describe the continuum from optimal blood sugar balance toward insulin resistance and full blown diabetes. Unfortunately, most of the eighty million people with pre-diabetes are well on their way to having the single biggest chronic disease in America. Pre-diabetes is simply a precursor to full-blown type 2 diabetes and carries all the same risks. It is a bit like cancer or heart disease in its early stages. So one out of every four Americans are already on this path and the numbers are getting worse!

Combined with smoking, "diabesity" causes nearly all the major health problems of the twenty-first century, including heart disease, stroke, dementia and cancer. I have to practically slap myself every time I see these numbers because to me they are hard to believe. They are scandalous, catastrophic and I don't use those words lightly! In fact, these numbers are so terrible that it is clear to me that our leaders and our people just simply do not understand the extent of the diabesity epidemic nor the implications for our future.

Epidemic No. 3: Alzheimer's

Alzheimer's and other forms of dementia are so closely linked to obesity and diabetes that they are increasingly referred to as Type 3 Diabetes.

It is very difficult to label one epidemic as worse than another but in my book, if you could, the Alzheimer's epidemic would fit the bill. I don't feel that way simply because I am pushing on in years, either. Alzheimer's disease

---

2   Mark Hyman, *Blood Sugar Solution* (New York: Little, Brown and Co., 2012)

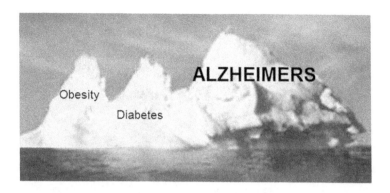

starts some <u>thirty years</u> before the first symptoms show! When I heard about this recently and then combined it with the problems of obesity and diabetes, I realized that we truly have a HUGE health problem looming in our relatively near future.

According to the Alzheimer's Association, Alzheimer's disease is now officially an epidemic in the United States. More than five million Americans have Alzheimer's today but alarmingly, though not surprisingly, based on what I revealed in the last paragraph, this total is expected to triple by 2050. Unfortunately, I have a big fear that this figure could be a lot worse unless we start to take serious proactive steps immediately.

According to Dr. Daniel Amen[3], another of my favorite authors and one of the world's leading authorities on the subject, "this is an illness you do not want to get". I am so concerned about the potential dangers of Alzheimer's that I have devoted Chapter 18 to the subject. However, don't wait for the Cavalry to arrive—take action yourself and get on a prevention program today!

Epidemic No. 4: The Inactivity Epidemic

The evidence supporting the health benefits of exercise is overwhelming. Regular exercise fundamentally changes your physiology including your musculoskeletal, circulatory, respiratory and nervous systems. This results in many positive health outcomes which are detailed later in Part 2 of this book. Exercise also has a profoundly positive effect on your ability to lose and then maintain your weight.

---

3   Dr. Daniel Amen, Brain Fit Life, http://www.MyBrainFitLife.com

Despite the overwhelming evidence of the benefits, the vast majority of Americans do not exercise enough. I believe that this is this fourth hidden epidemic which is in large part responsible for the other three: Obesity, Diabetes and Alzheimer's. I call this silent killer the **"Inactivity Epidemic"**.

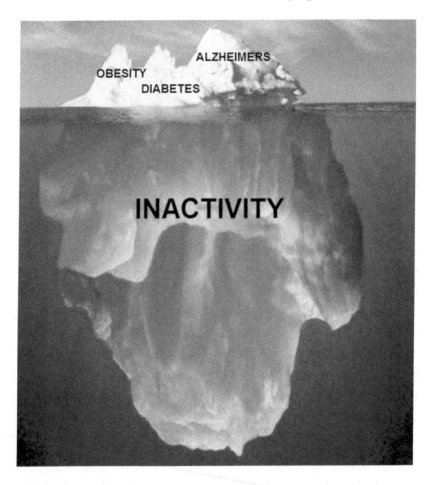

There are some serious risks associated with inactivity. Weight loss without exercise is very difficult to achieve and dieting will also negatively affect both your aerobic capacity and strength as your muscle mass reduces. In other words, it is impossible to maintain a healthy weight without exercise.

Research also shows that it is better to be overweight and exercise than to be normal weight and inactive. To put this another way, you can exercise and still be unhealthy but you simply cannot be healthy without exercise!

Reframe the Dialogue

Perhaps worst of all, inactivity seriously reduces your life expectancy. I believe that the risks of inactivity are not getting the attention they deserve. My use of the term "Inactivity Epidemic" may appear somewhat alarmist at first but when you consider what I have already said in this chapter and what I am going to say in the rest of Part 1, I hope you will agree with me that reframing the dialogue about inactivity and exercise is badly needed.

✗ Your "To Do" List

1. Simply recognize that as a nation we have some major health problems.
2. Ask yourself if you are part of the majority of Americans who do not exercise enough.
3. Acknowledge the importance of exercise; you cannot be healthy without it!

"The average American takes many years to get out of condition but expects to get back in condition in a few weeks; it's not going to happen!"
—Jim Kirwan

CHAPTER 2

THE VAST MAJORITY OF AMERICANS DO NOT EXERCISE ENOUGH

I believe that the vast majority of Americans do not exercise enough but I don't expect you to just accept my view without explaining why I believe this. According to the last reported figures in 2007, the Centers for Disease Control and Prevention (CDC) estimated that some 52% of Americans do not exercise enough[4]. Of these, 13.5% are inactive and the remainder do less than the recommended level. However, I believe the real figures are a lot worse because the recommended level to which they refer is too low!

To validate my hypothesis we need to have a good understanding of what enough exercise is. So we need to answer this important question:

---

4   Centers for Disease Control and Prevention. (2007). *Facts About Physical Activity.* http://www.cdc.gov

How much exercise is enough?

There are many different views about how long you should spend exercising and they are related to a second question—what kind or type of exercise should you do? I will give you very specific answers to both questions in Part 2, but for now let me address the general question of—how much exercise is enough?

Some current views are confusing, some are misleading and I hate to say it, but some are just plain wrong. Therefore, I believe you are entitled to get logical, easy to understand answers to the above question which are supported by scientific research. To help me do this I will refer, in turn, to three important sources as follows:

- The Official American View
- The Rest of the World View
- Great News from a Major Research Study

The Official American View

In 2008, the *Physical Activity Guidelines for Americans* were published. There is a general lack of familiarity among the folks about these *Guidelines*, which reinforces my belief that exercise is not getting the attention it deserves. Have you ever heard of the *Guidelines* or could you provide a quick summary of their key recommendations? Except for those who need to be familiar with the *Guidelines* as part of their job, I have never met anyone—not a single person—who could summarize their key messages.

The *Guidelines* were produced by the U.S. Department of Health and Human Services, based on a report submitted by the physical activity guidelines advisory committee, a group comprised of thirteen leading experts in the field of exercise science and public health. The *Guidelines* very clearly tell Americans that physical activity should be seen as an essential part of their lives:

> *"We know that sedentary behavior contributes to a host of chronic diseases and regular physical activity is an important component of an overall healthy lifestyle. There is strong evidence that physically active people have better health-related physical fitness and are at lower risk of developing many disabling medical conditions than inactive people."*

According to the report, the *Guidelines* were developed because we clearly know enough to recommend that all Americans should engage in regular physical activity to improve overall health and to reduce the risk of many health problems. While the primary target audience was policymakers and health professionals, I believe the *Guidelines* should be readily available to all. If you have time, I encourage you to read the full *Guidelines* report.[5]

The main idea behind the *Guidelines* is that regular physical activity, over months and years, can produce long-term health benefits. They very clearly state that being inactive or sedentary is unhealthy. **The biggest take-away from the *Guidelines* is that the more exercise you do, the greater your health benefits will be.**

For your convenience, I have reproduced a short summary of the *Guidelines'* key points, which apply to adults, below:

Summary—Physical Activity Guidelines 2008 (Adults 18-64)
Level 1: For Substantial Health Benefits Adults Should do:

At least 150 minutes of moderate intensity exercise a week

OR

75 minutes of vigorous intensity exercise

OR

An equivalent combination of moderate and vigorous exercise

PLUS

Muscle strengthening activities for all major muscle groups (legs, hips, back, chest, abdomen, shoulders and arms) on 2 or more days each week

Level 2: For Additional and More Extensive Health Benefits:

Increase to 300 minutes of moderate intensity exercise a week

OR

150 minutes of vigorous intensity exercise

OR

An equivalent combination of moderate and vigorous exercise

PLUS

---

5   U.S. Department of Health and Human Services. (2008). *2008 Physical Activity Guidelines for Americans.* Retrieved from http://www.health.gov/paguidelines

Muscle strengthening activities for all major muscle groups (legs, hips, back, chest, abdomen, shoulders and arms) on 2 or more days a week

Level 3: Additional Health Benefits are Gained by Engaging in Physical Activity Beyond this Amount.

The statement about Level 3 is both clear and vague at the same time. Sounds a bit Irish, I know, but hey, I'm Irish so I can say that. Clearly, "Additional Health Benefits" are gained by engaging in exercise beyond Level 2, but it is vague about the amount. However, when read in conjunction with pages ten and eleven, it becomes a lot clearer. On page ten, when talking about premature death, the *Guidelines* say:

> *"Strong scientific evidence shows that physical activity reduces the risk of premature death from the leading causes of death. The effect is remarkable....*
>
> *Only a few lifestyle choices have as large an effect on mortality as physical activity. It has been estimated that people who are physically active for approximately seven hours a week have a 40% lower risk of dying early than those who are active for less than thirty minutes a week."*

They support this text by including a graph on page eleven, which is reproduced below.

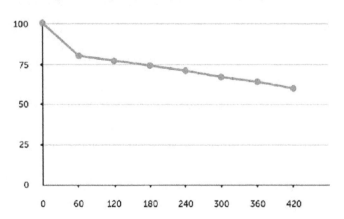

Minutes per Week of Moderate or Vigorous Intensity Exercise

The Risk of Dying Prematurely Declines as People Become More Physically Active

The Risk of Dying Prematurely Declines as People Become Physically Active

The graph shows that the risk of dying prematurely declines as the amount of physical activity increases, with the greatest decline of 40% occurring when a person does four hundred twenty minutes (seven hours) of exercise a week.

New Guidelines

The *Guidelines* are a little dated at this stage though they are currently under review. There was a Midcourse Report released in 2013 called *Strategies to Increase Physical Activity Among Youth*. The Midcourse Report Infographic is reproduced below and I wish to highlight two clear messages:

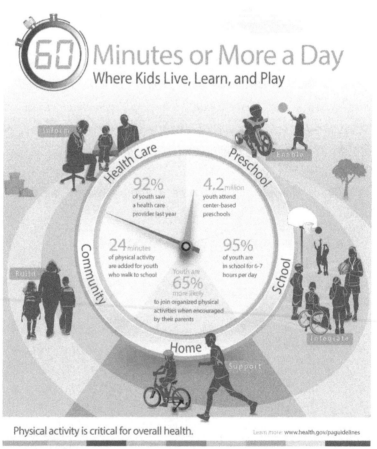

The headline says, "**60 Minutes or More a Day.**" While this refers to youth, I can think of no good reason why it shouldn't apply to adults, too.

At the bottom it says, "**Physical Activity is Critical for Overall Health.**" This is the first time I have heard an official reference to exercise as critical. If this is true, why do we not pay much greater attention to exercise than we do?

Conclusions about the Official American View

1. The *Physical Activity Guidelines for Americans* clearly demonstrate that the benefits of physical activity increase the more time you spend exercising, with the greatest benefit occurring at seven hours a week. They do not consider what happens beyond this point.

2. If you are inactive or exercise less than two hours a week, Level 1 is a good starting point. However, it is only a stepping stone on the way to the level of physical activity required to maximize your life expectancy and quality of life.

3. Some exercise is better than no exercise at all. However, the emphasis on the minimum recommended level of exercise (Level 1) as an "acceptable level" of exercise helps to explain why the vast majority of Americans do not exercise enough and why we have what I call the "Inactivity Epidemic". Clearly we need to exercise more!

4. I believe this is done because the authors fear many folks would be put off by the much more demanding optimum level of seven hours. They just want you to get started, hoping you will be converted later. While this is a reasonable stance, without effective follow-through and clear communication of the ultimate goal, the vast majority of Americans will continue to significantly under-exercise and experience all the negative consequences that entails.

5. Unfortunately, what I call the "Inactivity Epidemic" puts the health of many Americans at unnecessary risk. Very little progress has been made in meeting the objectives of the *Guidelines*.

6. Exercise is critical for overall health and thus we should see it as a high priority in our lives.

If you are thinking right now that you could never do seven hours of exercise a week, please don't worry because that is in the future. For now, focus on the present and start at Level 1. You can definitely do that!

The *Guidelines* clearly demonstrate that increasing the amount of exercise you do results in further reduction in the risk of cardiovascular disease. Also, there is strong scientific evidence that exercise will help you to maintain a stable weight over time. According to the *Guidelines*:

> *"The bottom line is that the health benefits of physical activity far outweigh the risks of adverse events for almost everyone."*

Validation of My Hypothesis

Level 1 is the minimum recommended level of physical activity. Revisit the summary of the *Guidelines* above and note the reference to the words "at least" in Level 1. The reason the CDC figure of 52% is too low is because it is based on the minimum recommended weekly exercise. What would the figure be if it was based on Level 2 or 3 or the optimum level of 7 hours a week? I believe this validates my hypothesis that **the vast majority of Americans do not exercise enough.** My hypothesis is supported by what the rest of the world says and by great news from a major research study. Both are described below.

What the Rest of the World Says

In 2010 the World Health Organization published their ***Global Recommendations on Physical Activity for Health***. There is significant overlap with the 2008 *Physical Activity Guidelines for Americans*.

The report highlights that physical inactivity is now the fourth leading risk factor for global mortality and that physical inactivity levels are rising all across the world with major implications for the general health of the population worldwide.

The leading risk factors for global mortality are ranked as follows:

1st	High Blood Pressure	13%
2nd	Tobacco Usage	9%
3rd	High Blood Glucose	6%
4th	Physical Inactivity	6%
5th	Overweight and Obesity	5%

When you consider these leading risk factors together, they account for 39% of global mortality. What is striking is the fact that all of these top five risk factors are interrelated. While physical inactivity only accounts for 6%, there is a very strong correlation between it and the other four factors.

Physical Inactivity facilitates high blood pressure, high blood glucose, as well as being overweight and obese. The link with tobacco may not be as direct but there is some evidence that exercise does help smoking cessation. I also personally believe that active people, who experience all the associated positive health consequences of exercise, are less likely to smoke than people who lead more sedentary lifestyles.

So the World Health Organization Report really confirms that there is an "Inactivity Epidemic" not just in America, but all across the world. The good news again, however, is that simply switching from being inactive to being active will have a significant positive effect on your health and life expectancy!

Great News from a Major Research Study

The 2008 *Physical Activity Guidelines for Americans* demonstrate that the **benefits of physical activity increase the more time you spend exercising**, with the greatest benefit occurring at seven hours a week.

There is a major research study which was completed in 2012[6] that examined the association between leisure time physical activity and mortality, in pooled data from six studies in the National Cancer Institute Cohort Consortium, comprising 654,827 individuals, from twenty-one to ninety years of age.

Physical activity is shown in minutes with a focus on moderate and vigorous intensity, consistent with the 2008 *Physical Activity Guidelines for Americans* and

---

6   Moore, S. PLOS Medicine. (2012). *Leisure Time Physical Activity of Moderate to Vigorous Intensity and Mortality: A Large Pooled Cohort Analysis.*

the 2010 World Health Organization Guidelines. The findings are summarized in the following graph:

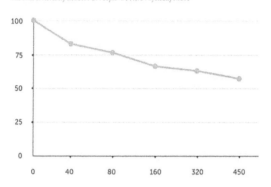

(Source: PLOS Medicine—Stephen C. Moore)

Major Conclusions From Study

The study's findings reinforce the public health message that a physically active lifestyle is important for increasing life expectancy. The greatest gain in life expectancy takes place at a physical activity level of four hundred fifty minutes (or 7 ½ hours) of exercise per week or above. The highest reduction in the risk of mortality achieved (41%) is almost identical to the findings of the 2008 *Physical Activity Guidelines for Americans*.

Some Other Important Findings of Study

There were 654,827 participants in the 2012 study and they had some interesting characteristics:

1. 49% were between sixty and seventy years of age, with 9% aged seventy or over. This proves that you are never too old for exercise.
2. 48% were former smokers with only 11% current smokers. This suggests that exercise helps many folks stop and stay off smoking.
3. 53% were overweight (BMI > 24.9) with 12% of these obese (BMI 30). This proves that you are never too heavy for exercise.
4. 53% were women, 97% were white and 41% were college graduates.

BAD News: The study shows that when combined, a lack of activity and a high Body Mass Index (BMI) result in premature death. A BMI of 35+ (Obese Class 2+) was associated with ***seven years of life lost***, compared to meeting recommended activity levels and being normal weight. By comparison, long-term cigarette smoking reduces life expectancy by approximately ten years.

GOOD News: Another important finding is that physically active Class 1 Obese (BMI 30–34.9) participants live longer than normal weight participants who are inactive. This finding should convince currently inactive and/or overweight people that exercise is definitely worthwhile, not only for health benefits but also for increased life expectancy. Unfortunately, this finding does not apply to physically active Class 2 obese participants so they have to reduce their weight to get this benefit.

✗ Your "To Do" List

1. Acknowledge that the more exercise you do, the greater your health benefits will be.
2. If you are inactive, start exercising and work your way up to Level 1, but remember—this is only a stepping stone on the road to the optimum level.
3. Accept that exercise is critical for your overall health and thus it should be a high priority in your life.
4. If you are overweight, start exercise today and remember that if you are active you will live longer than people who are normal weight, but inactive.

"Fitness is not about being better than someone else;
it's about being better than you used to be!"
—Unknown

CHAPTER 3

MAJOR CAUSES OF THE INACTIVITY EPIDEMIC

Our politicians fight over the size of the national debt and the budget deficit. They argue about the fiscal cliff and the debt ceiling. Healthcare is another major political football but I doubt that the politicians have any idea of what is coming down the tracks.

If we do not get our act together quickly, the cumulative cost of the four epidemics I have described and all the associated health problems will have a major negative effect on an already seriously strained healthcare and economic system. Furthermore, it could have a devastating effect on the social fabric of the nation.

This raises some important questions: how has this happened and how did we get to this point? Why are these health problems, and inactivity in particular, such low priorities?

How has this happened?

Humans are hardwired to be physically active and we have been for a very long time. The fact is our genes have simply been unable to respond to the speed of the changes that have taken place in the last thirty or forty years. Our bodies are simply not ready for life in the twenty-first century; nature prepared us for a totally different existence.

Without having to go back too far, we find that our ancestors lived a completely different life. If my father, who died in 1975, was to somehow return to Planet Earth today, he would probably suffer another massive heart attack from the shock!

If you analyze how the average human spends his time today you will quickly see how different it is. We travel everywhere in cars, buses and trains. We sit at desks all day whether we are at work, at school or college. We also spend most of our free time sitting, watching TV, playing computer games and on our wide variety of mobile devices. We eat regularly at restaurants where the portions are too big, and far too often at fast food restaurants. We also eat too much processed and take-out food at home.

Seven Major Causes

The Inactivity Epidemic has taken about thirty or forty years to develop by stealth and from my perspective, regretfully, it is not going away any time soon. There are many reasons for this, so I have identified seven major causes which I will review, one by one, starting with what is probably the primary driver of the Inactivity Epidemic.

1. Change

The changes that have taken place in my lifetime are amazing. I grew up in the sixties in Ireland, when television was black and white and not very exciting. When I started working in the seventies, typewriters, secretaries and typing pools were all the rage. To my kids, this sounds like the dark ages.

Unfortunately, this change and progress, which are otherwise very good, have produced some decidedly negative byproducts. The average level of our daily physical activity has seriously suffered because of positive developments elsewhere. Think about remote controls, computer games, online movies, elevators, escalators, fast food drive-thrus and online shopping, to name just a few.

Today we also spend a huge amount of our time sitting! This applies to adults and children alike, whether we are at work or at play. When I was a young teenager, I spent nearly all my spare time outdoors "playing"; the activities ranged from impromptu soccer and tip rugby matches to simple games of hide and seek. There were no computer games, online movies or smart phones, and I was only allowed to watch television on weekend nights. To be honest, even then playing with my pals won out most of the time!

Unplanned Exercise

Everything we do from when we get up in the morning to when we go to bed at night includes some kind of unplanned exercise. Unplanned exercise excludes all planned exercise, such as going for a thirty minute walk, a four mile run, a fifteen hundred meter swim, a twenty mile bike ride or an aerobics class at the gym. There may not be much unplanned exercise attached to sitting in your car or at your desk at work or at home watching television, but it is there! Unplanned exercise is sometimes called "Baseline" exercise and I will deal with this in much greater detail in Chapter 9: What Type of Exercise Should You Do?

Change and progress have significantly reduced the amount of unplanned exercise we do in a day. I can vividly remember when I was a boy, playing in the back yard and my mum interrupting our game of football (soccer or tip rugby). She would carry this big basket of laundry out into the middle of the yard and then hang wet sheets, towels and clothes on a line with pegs. Think of all the baseline exercise involved in her activity, which was repeated a few hours later when she came back to collect the dry clothes.

I can also remember during summer vacations, my older sister Margaret and I would get on our bikes early in the morning and ride three miles to a popular outdoor pool called Blackrock Baths on the coast, south of Dublin (see photo). The pool was filled every other day by the incoming tide and we spent our days swimming and running around the pool, jumping and diving off the boards and into the surrounding sea. In the evening, we got back on our bikes and rode the three miles uphill, home. Looking back now, we were incredibly active compared to kids today. I often joke that we did the equivalent of a

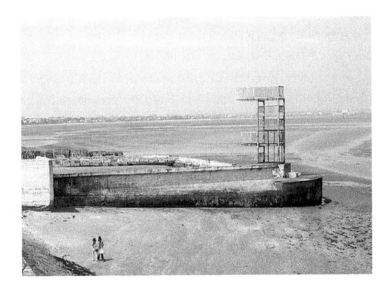

triathlon every day! At the time, though, we were just having fun and never thought about it as exercise.

Over the years, this type of unplanned exercise has been decimated. These changes are a huge problem and as such are a major cause of the Inactivity Epidemic. Even the outdoor pool of my childhood which gave me so many happy memories is gone!

Planned Exercise

Having discussed unplanned exercise, let's now look at planned exercise. The problem I have with planned exercise is different because this hasn't changed very much over the years.

Question: Why do so many adults retire from exercise in their thirties?

Many adults stop playing sports or games, their planned exercise, once they are out of school or college and never get started again. While this in itself is cause for concern, thankfully many continue to play sports well into their thirties until they "retire" and then stop.

For most competitive team sports, the vast majority of adults retire in their early thirties. Some may stop earlier and some may retire later, but this is fair enough in physically active team sports such as football, soccer, hockey, rugby and lacrosse, where the majority of participants are in their late teens and twenties.

It is also reasonable to stop competitive individual sports such as track and field, swimming, boxing and wrestling, because these sports do take a lot out of you and as you get older, it is difficult to compete with much younger athletes. There are some individual sports, however, where it is possible to continue well beyond your thirties, such as tennis or show jumping.

I played rugby when I was younger and I have no desire to play the full-blown version of that sport at my age now. Despite this, I sometimes wish I could play tip rugby again, which relies on speed and endurance without the brute force.

Why, then, do so many adults stop participating in exercise completely? That is what my dad did when he stopped playing rugby and I am sure this lack of exercise for the remaining fifteen years of his life played a big part in his premature death.

I also think, at least for males, that the fact that we can no longer play the way we could when we were younger is an important factor. Our pride is not able to handle the idea of playing at a lower standard or level than we once did. I see this all the time in running and it stops many men from ever getting started.

We don't have to be super athletes all our lives, assuming we ever were in the first place. This is a very important concept to grasp when exercise and physical activity return to their rightful place on your list of priorities.

2. Convenience

As all these changes in our lifestyle have occurred, we have also developed a culture of convenience. We want everything to be quick and easy and we want it now. This culture of convenience has unfortunately spilled over into physical activity.

Do you wait for the elevator or do you take the stairs? Escalators, which are now everywhere, were introduced to help you walk from point A to point B more quickly. However, most people now stand on escalators. I was in the Atlanta airport recently and in a hurry to get from one terminal to another. I missed a train because everyone on the escalator was standing and I couldn't pass and there are no stairs available in that part of the airport. As things turned out, it didn't really matter because I caught my plane!

Exercise increasingly gets a bad rap, even from within the fitness community. According to some fitness experts, certain types of exercise, especially cardio, are boring as well as a waste of time. These experts are usually promoting a product which treats exercise as a "convenience" to be completed in a short timeframe. This is unfortunately an attractive proposition to an increasing number of people.

Don't misunderstand me, I am all for change and progress, especially when they lead to new and progressive ways of doing things. But we need to be aware of the potential consequences of this progress and adapt our behavior to accommodate the positive developments while minimizing potential negative side effects, especially with regard to our health.

Sitting the New Smoking

Some more bad news in our culture of convenience is that our lives have evolved to the point where most of us spend too much of our non-sleeping time just sitting. There is probably an inverse relationship between the amount of time you spend sitting and your overall health. In other words, the more time you spend sitting the worse your health is likely to be. All the time you spend sitting, behind your steering wheel, slumped over your laptop or PC or sprawled out on your couch watching television, is linked to an increased risk of heart disease, diabetes and cancer. This has progressed to such an extent that sitting is increasingly being referred to as the "New Smoking".

Incredibly, there is still more bad news. Even if you exercise regularly for, say an average of an hour a day, which is the optimum level of seven hours a week, you are still at risk if you are sedentary the rest of the time.

In a study published in the *International Journal of Behavioral Nutrition and Physical Activity* in 2012, researchers reported that active people sit just as much as inactive folks, averaging sixty-four hours a week, or slightly over nine hours of sitting each day. Unless you are active throughout the day you are effectively an "active Couch Potato", a phrase coined by Australian researcher Genevieve Healy, Ph.D. (University of Queensland).

I will explore this issue further in Part 2 when we discuss "Baseline" exercise.

3. Consensus

We really need a consensus about the importance of exercise and this should be clearly communicated to everyone. There are some fundamental things about exercise that we could and should all agree on. Unfortunately, this is probably "pie in the sky" but I really believe that we could do a much better job communicating important information such as the *Physical Activity Guidelines for Americans.*

The *Guidelines* in their current format may not be perfect but they could fill the void created by the current lack of consensus among fitness experts, a lack of consensus which has led to inertia and hindered much needed progress.

Consensus about the positive benefits of exercise and the dangers of inactivity would lead to far less confusion and a more active population.

4. Confusion

The lack of consensus among fitness experts leads to confusion among the folks about some fundamental issues regarding exercise. Depending on whom you ask, you will get different answers to key questions such as, "What kind of exercise should you do?" and "How much time should you spend exercising?"

This means people don't know who or what to believe and this is not a helpful situation to have. Conflicting, misleading and often inaccurate information makes it very difficult to know who is telling the truth. It is a minefield out there; who knows what to believe anymore and this confusion is not confined simply to exercise, either.

We need to keep up with developments in science where the goalposts keep changing. Is fat good for us or bad? Is high cholesterol bad? Is cardio good for us or not? Also, we are expected to be able to interpret and see beyond advertisements produced by the vast marketing budgets of corporate America, which may not always tell the truth. Consider the following examples:

- A major soft drink company has recently rolled out an advertising campaign disguised as a public service announcement to fight obesity.
- A diet called "The Food Lovers Fat Loss System" claims to allow you to "eat all your favorite foods at every meal and reduce your waistline".

- Several exercise advertisements and infomercials claim to provide the magic pill or silver bullet and they all promote what I call the "less is more" approach.

Each of these are examples of companies getting away with what is, at best, confusing and misleading information to the consumer.

5. Cardio

Perhaps the greatest lack of consensus among fitness experts which leads to confusion among the general population applies to cardio or aerobic exercise. While some say it is good, many others say it is bad. The reality is that when fitness experts discuss "cardio", they are seldom talking about the same thing and are usually using the term in a way that suits their current needs, such as helping to sell a product. Typically, when referring to cardio, they mean exercising for a long time, thirty minutes or more, at the same slow pace on a treadmill or exercise machine. In my experience over many years, there are very few people who actually exercise this way.

I believe there is a definitive answer to this question - Is cardio good or bad for you? According to the American College of Sports Medicine:

"Cardio or cardiovascular exercise is any activity that increases heart rate and respiration while using large muscle groups repetitively and rhythmically. Progressively challenging your most vital life support network, cardio can improve function and performance of your heart, lungs and circulatory system."

Applying that definition, I think it is reasonable to assume that cardio is good for you. In my opinion, the most important words here are *"progressively challenging"*. With these words included in the definition, I believe that there really should be no doubt about it. So let me be clear:

Cardio is good for you!

However, let me also be clear that cardio or aerobic exercise alone is not always the BEST exercise for you. Your exercise program should be progressive in nature, which means that you should gradually increase the intensity of your workouts, as well as introduce muscle strengthening into your training. However the bottom line is that cardio is good for you and this is true with very few exceptions, which the vast majority of you reading this book don't need to worry about.

I will deal with the subject of cardio or aerobic exercise in much greater detail in Part 2, including 10 reasons why you must include it in your exercise regimen.

6. Calories

It is clear from our major health epidemics that far too many Americans are consuming too many calories. There are many reasons for this but I believe it is partly because there is a general lack of knowledge and understanding of the direct link between calories and exercise.

I have produced an easy-to-follow graph which shows the relationship between exercise and calories. As I want to keep this message simple and easy to understand, the graph is not intended to be precise, so I have ignored some other variables such as the quality of your calories, the intensity of your exercise and your metabolism.

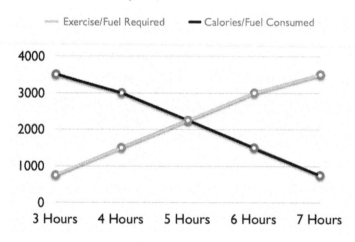

The Relationship Between Exercise and Calories

The calories we consume give us the energy we need to go about our daily lives, including exercise. The vertical axis measures the amount of fuel or calories, while the horizontal axis measures time in hours. If you look at exercise, you can see that the more exercise you do the more time it takes and the more fuel or calories you require. Conversely, the less exercise you do the fewer calories you require. So if you consume more calories than you need for the amount of exercise you do you will increase weight. Likewise, if you consume fewer calories than you need you will lose weight. Consequently, you need to find a balance between these two positions.

Let's consider an example. If you exercise around the minimum recommended level of three hours a week at a moderate intensity, you will not be exercising enough to lose weight and unless you reduce your calories your weight will likely increase.

On the other hand, as you progress and your exercise time and intensity increase, you require more calories. Therefore, it becomes much easier to lose weight at this exercise level, so long as you control your calorie intake. The bottom line is this—if you want to lose weight, you need to progressively increase the amount of exercise you do with a corresponding controlled calorie intake. You must be patient, however, because this does not and cannot happen overnight. This is a gradual process that is much better than short-term dieting because it leads to a much more sustained, healthy lifestyle over the long term.

7. Control

I mentioned earlier that healthcare has become a major political football in America. While the politicians are debating legitimate healthcare issues they seem to continually and consistently pay lip service to the major health problems facing the nation. While I don't think they fully understand the extent of the problems we face, I believe there are other forces in play, such as the interests of the food and pharmaceutical industries. Accordingly, you have to take control of your own life as I cannot see anyone else doing this for you.

Two Groups

Just like the political system in America, there are essentially only two groups of people when it comes to exercise. However, unlike politics where the group with the greatest support wins, in the realm of exercise it is the very small minority that are the winners. And unfortunately, the much larger group, who don't exercise enough, are the losers. The big challenge facing America today is how to get more people to switch from the majority group to the minority so that in time the minority can become the majority.

With many years of experience and seeing literally thousands of people make the switch, I have a solution which is easy to explain and understand. However, having said that, putting this solution into practice is much easier said than done. Let me explain.

Many people who are inactive or don't exercise enough live this way because they believe that they don't really like or enjoy exercise. This is based on their actual experience, because whenever they try to get started again they find it very difficult and certainly not much fun. Unfortunately, based on this experience alone, the vast majority of people quit exercising and fall by the wayside. It is not an exaggeration to say that having tried it before, perhaps many times, they now hate this process!

The Promised Land

Yet, what about those who persevere and make it to the Promised Land? Nearly every single woman or man who makes it that far will tell you that it was tough, really tough, but they are so glad they stuck it out. That is not the only interesting thing that happens to them, however. As if by some divine intervention, they are converted into the fold of "exercise junkies", regardless of whether it is running, cycling, swimming, etc. They are now addicted to exercise and when they look back, usually after about a year, to where they came from, they wonder how it took them so long to make the switch to their new active lifestyle.

I'm sure you are familiar with the popular television program called *The Biggest Loser*. Think of the participants at the start and then compare that to the end. Chalk and cheese! Because it is for television, the process is concentrated into a shorter time but the same principle applies; the participants go from hatred to addicted in around five or six months!

If you accept that what I have just described is indeed the solution for many, though unfortunately still a small minority of people, then with similar effort, perseverance and will, it can be the solution for you. All you have to do now is take control!

Ultimately, you are in control of your own destiny. You can either make good decisions to improve your health and with it your life expectancy and the quality of your life, or you can make bad decisions.

✗ Your "To Do" List

1. Understand the changes that have taken place to unplanned exercise and adapt your behavior.
2. Accept that you don't have to be a superstar when it comes to planned exercise and if appropriate start again.
3. Cardio or aerobic exercise is good for you, so make sure you include it in your exercise program.
4. If you want to lose weight, progressively increase your exercise with a corresponding controlled calorie intake.
5. You are in control of your destiny! Make the right decisions to improve your life expectancy and quality of life.

*"My suggestion would be to walk away from the 90%
who don't and join the 10% who do."*
—Jim Rohn

CHAPTER 4

WHAT ARE YOU GOING TO DO?

L ife expectancy is a term used to predict how long we can expect to live based on historical data. Throughout the twentieth century and the early years of the twenty-first century our life expectancy continued to increase largely due to advances in medicine. However, this positive trend may not continue for much longer.

There is increasing evidence for a likely decline in life expectancy for future generations, at least in the near future. There is another measure we also need to be aware of and which we need to pay more attention to. Getting older may not be an option, but what about the quality of our lives? Let's take a look at life expectancy, then, from both a quantitative and a qualitative perspective.

Life Expectancy—Quantity

The traditional way to talk about life expectancy is to refer to life expectancy from birth. However, this is not a good measure for folks in their thirties, forties or fifties. In fact, it is not really a good measure at all, once you have survived your early childhood. As you can see from the table below, the longer you survive, the greater your life expectancy.

Life Expectancy (2009)	Males	Females	All
At Birth	76.0	80.9	78.5
At 65 Years	82.6	85.3	84.2
Source: US Dept. of Health and Human Services			

I have chosen sixty-five in the table above for two reasons. First, the latest figures available from 2009 are only available for sixty-five and from birth. Second, it is an important milestone we all aspire to achieve. While sixty-five has been our traditional age of "retirement" the latest life expectancy figures clearly demonstrate that this is one tradition that is very much out of date.

In the above table, the average male can expect to live close to eighty-three years; that's an additional eighteen years, at age sixty-five. The average female can expect to live to just over eighty-five; that's an additional twenty years.

Of course by definition, all life expectancy figures are average figures which means they include everyone, in bad health as well as good. So your life expectancy could be lower or higher than the average depending on your personal circumstances. Consequently, you can see that aspiring to reach ninety, ninety-five or even a hundred years old is no longer unrealistic.

Life Expectancy—Quality

Of course some of you will say, "What's the point of aspiring to reach one hundred if your quality of life is horrible?" That is a valid point. Extension of life doesn't necessarily translate into the extension of healthy life and this principle applies to all ages. Accordingly, there is another measure which adjusts life expectancy to account for the years expected to be lived with limitations and this is called "Active Life Expectancy".

As you can see from the table below, expected years of life free from chronic activity limitations are not quite as attractive.

Active Life Expectancy (2006)	Males	Females	All
At Birth	65.1	68.4	66.7
At 65 Years	76.6	77.6	77.2
Source: US Dept. of Health and Human Services			

In this table the average male at age sixty-five can expect to live less than twelve years free from chronic activity limitations. The average female can expect to live under thirteen years. If you compare the Active Life Expectancy with the Life Expectancy figures at sixty-five you will find the following differences:

	Males	Females	All
Life Expectancy at 65 Years	82.6	85.3	84.2
Active Life Expectancy	76.6	77.6	77.2
Years with Chronic Activity Limitations	6.0	7.7	7.0

The average male has six years with chronic activity limitations while the average female has just under eight years. This is a long time and the overall figure of seven years represents 36.5% which is over a third of your expected remaining time, once you reach sixty-five.

Is Life Expectancy just a throw of the dice?

At the end of the last chapter, I said that you can either make good decisions to improve your health or you can make bad ones. In referring to health, I was referring to both your quality of life and your life expectancy. So is your life expectancy and quality of life just a throw of the dice or is it something that you can proactively manage?

If our collective behavior regarding health is anything to go by, then you could simply conclude that most people believe it is just a throw of the dice. However, I don't think it is as simple as that. There is no doubt that heredity is an important factor and that the hand of cards you were dealt can and does influence your life expectancy. But just how influential is it and can you do anything to influence your cards or load the dice in your favor?

I believe you can *dramatically* increase your life expectancy and improve the quality of your life by the actions you take now. I'd better be right, because I wasn't dealt a great hand. As you already know my dad died from a sudden heart attack at forty-seven. He suffered from angina which is the most common symptom of coronary artery disease. Angina is caused when blood flow to an area of the heart is decreased, impairing the delivery of oxygen and vital nutrients to the heart muscle cells. Dad was on angina medication, which clearly didn't work. He didn't smoke, very seldom drank and had a reasonable diet, although he was probably ten or fifteen pounds overweight. And, as you already know, he didn't exercise!

My mum died at sixty-nine from cancer, though the disease had been part of her life for about 5 years. Unlike dad who died suddenly, she left home one day to go into the hospital for further treatment, hopeful that she would get better. Of course, my sisters and I knew differently, and as we had suspected, she deteriorated very quickly, dying only a few weeks later. Like dad, mum was a non-smoker, seldom drank, had a pretty good diet (especially after dad died) and was a normal weight. However, she didn't exercise either!

I realize that heredity is an important factor and that there are no guarantees that your actions will lead to a long, high quality life. However, I believe your actions will influence things one way or the other. If you want to add fuel to the fire of your hand of cards, then you should do the following:

- Smoke
- Eat lots of junk food
- Drink lots of sodas and alcohol
- Do very little or no exercise
- Become overweight and obese

On the other hand, I believe that there are many positive actions you can take to stack the deck of cards in your favor including:

- Eat good food and minimize the junk
- Drink plenty of water and minimize the caffeine
- Limit your alcohol intake (I only drink red wine and the occasional beer)
- Exercise seven hours a week, including muscle strengthening and higher intensity
- Maintain a healthy weight

Think about it this way—if you were the owner of an expensive race horse, how would you treat it?

But what do you believe?

To help you answer this very broad, open-ended question, let me try to break it down by asking you four questions which I regularly use in talks about this subject.

Question 1: What is the most important thing in your life?

Another general question, I know, but this gets you involved and thinking about what is important to you. Not surprisingly, to me at any rate, the vast majority answer family and/or health. Occasionally I get a specific answer relating to the person's career or hobby, but when challenged, the person nearly always agrees that these are short-term priorities. Still, family and/or health is somewhat vague so I follow up with my second question.

Question 2: What do you mean by family and/or health; what do you *really* want?

The answer I get is nearly always you want to live a long, happy, high quality life where you are able to do the things you like doing with the ones you love. Roughly translated this means that most people do actually believe that life expectancy and the quality of their lives are important. This leads me to ask my third question.

Question 3: Is there congruence between what you want and what you do?

When faced with this question, most people will admit that there is a gap— often a very wide one—between what they *want* and what they *do*. I'm talking about their actions on a daily, weekly, monthly and yearly basis. This leads me to ask my fourth question.

Question 4: Are you on the slippery slope of aging?

I found the term "slippery slope" in one of my favorite books, *Younger Next Year*, written by Chris Crowley and Harry S. Lodge, M.D. I like this term so much that I have reproduced it below. This is what the slippery slope of aging looks like for most people, taking chronic activity limitations into account.

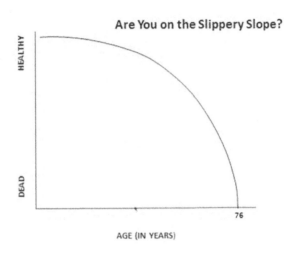

"Natural aging" today wrongly assumes that injury, illness and disease are the norm—the normal consequences of aging. For the vast majority of Americans this aging process probably starts in their thirties when many of us "retire" from exercise and begin to lose muscle mass and put on weight. We are more often than not over-nourished, over-medicated, physically and sometimes mentally inactive. This inactivity, which I call the "Inactivity Epidemic", is a major cause of disease and death!

As we get older, some changes occur which are unavoidable. For example, we need reading glasses as the lens of the eye thickens, stiffens and becomes less able to focus on close objects. While this may be considered normal aging, it doesn't mean that we have to accept everything that happens as normal.

This "normal aging" process is reinforced by normal retirement at age sixty-five, which is another very serious challenge facing the US and indeed the world as a whole. The notion of retirement at sixty-five made sense fifty or sixty years ago but as I mentioned earlier, it no longer makes sense today, where the average life expectancy of a sixty-five year old is nearly eighty-five.

Unfortunately, the concept of normal retirement at sixty-five also reinforces the belief in many people's minds that they have reached "old age". If I had never left the Bank of Ireland (my first full-time job), like many of my contemporaries, I would be due to retire after forty-five years of service. That would be less than four years from now in 2018. Scary for me if not for you!

Our health and pension systems are unsustainable as we never anticipated funding all kinds of additional age-related health costs, along with an average of some 20 years of retirement. We are sitting on a potential health and financial time bomb unless we do something about it and quickly!

Get Off the Slippery Slope

In the meantime, you don't have to accept this as "normal aging". Thankfully, there is an alternative to the slippery slope.

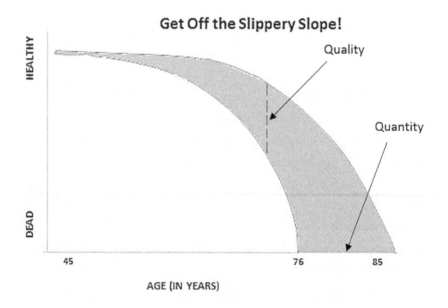

The above graph merges the message in *Younger Next Year* with the quantitative and qualitative approach to life expectancy we explored earlier. The alternative to "normal" aging is to get off the slippery slope by taking action. You can do this at any time; you just have to decide to do it and then, like the Nike ad says, just do it!

I know it sounds easy but it's not! It is, however, very doable and many have taken this path before. You can decide to take action today to get off the slippery slope and change your life's path or journey forever. At the same time, you can increase both the quantity and quality of your life, regardless of your age, weight or current fitness level. While there are no guarantees, your future actions will load the dice in your favor and will have a very positive influence on your outcome.

If my dad was alive today, he would be eighty-six years old. That's just one year more than the average life expectancy—not an unreasonable target. Instead, he lost thirty-nine years of his life. Please do not let this happen to you!

So what are you going to do?

X Your "To Do" List

1. Do you believe your life expectancy is just a throw of the dice? Make sure you answer the four questions in this chapter.
2. Don't accept "normal aging"; decide to get off the slippery slope.
3. While there are no guarantees, decide on what you would like your life expectancy to be.
4. Decide to take action to achieve your twin objectives of increased life expectancy with a significantly improved quality of life.

> *"The normal experience of the body and its aging is a*
> *conditioned response — a habit of thinking and behavior.*
> *By changing your habits of thinking and behavior, you can*
> *change the experience of your body and its aging."*
> **—Deepak Chopra**

YOUR FOUR KEY DRIVERS OF SUCCESS

Y ou too can decide to get off the slippery slope and change your life. Anyone can and it is never too late. I truly believe that you can do this if you want to, but you really have to want it.

What do you have to do?

There are a number of things that you have to do if you want to succeed and have a long, happy, high quality life. There are four key ingredients which I call Your Four Key Drivers of Success, as follows:

1. Exercise
2. The X Factor
3. Knowledge
4. Nutrition

Chapter 5 is the shortest chapter in the book but it is arguably the most important of all. You need to understand how each driver works but most important of all is that they work together in a holistic way. When all four drivers are working effectively together, you can turbo-charge your success. For example, you can lose weight without exercise but will it be effective in the long run? The rest of the book is devoted to the four key drivers. As we discuss each driver, please remember that for best results they should not be considered in isolation.

1. Exercise: Your first key driver is exercise and you won't be surprised to hear that I believe that exercise is a critical driver and the "secret sauce" to a long, high quality life. Accordingly, Part 2, the next part of the book, is devoted entirely to the importance of exercise.

2. The X Factor: Your second key driver works very closely alongside exercise and together these two critical drivers led to the book's title—*The eXercise Factor*. If you have it you are very likely to succeed but if you don't I am afraid you are doomed to fail. I call this the X Factor and if you don't know what it is yet, I would like you to think about it before you turn to Part 3 where it is revealed. With the X Factor you will be all set to ease into the best shape of your life.

3. Knowledge: Your third key driver is knowledge. I am referring to knowledge about each of the other ingredients, but especially about your health. I have thought long and hard about whether I should include knowledge as one of my drivers, as I do not want to appear disrespectful or condescending and I certainly don't want to insult anyone. However, because I feel so strongly about the importance of knowledge, Part 4 is devoted to key subjects not included elsewhere in the book.

4. Nutrition: Your fourth key driver is nutrition. You need to educate yourself and then implement healthy eating and drinking initiatives on an ongoing basis. If you could eliminate or significantly cut the junk from your diet you would be well on your way. There is a chapter about nutrition in Part 4.

X Your "To Do" List

1. Decide to make exercise your secret sauce and a high priority for the rest of your life.
2. You need to have the X Factor to succeed. If you have it, great! If you haven't, you must decide how you are going to get it.

3. Decide to increase your knowledge about exercise, nutrition and the X Factor but especially about your health.

4. Decide to implement a healthy nutrition initiative; eat and drink healthily for the rest of your life.

"Warning! Daily exercise and healthy eating
lead to increased awesomeness!"
—Unknown

PART 2

EXERCISE—THE SECRET SAUCE TO A GREAT LIFE

INTRODUCTION TO PART 2

In Part 2 of *The eXercise Factor*, I set out my case for why I believe exercise really is the secret sauce to a long, high quality life. However, I want to start by confronting some of the greatest obstacles which can get in your way, because we know that the vast majority of people don't exercise enough even though there is overwhelming evidence that inactivity is very bad indeed.

In **Chapter 6**, I explain that there are Thirteen Obstacles to Exercise which are stopping many people like you in their tracks. I hope my comments will help you overcome what may be stopping you from exercising.

In **Chapter 7**, I explain why and how you can make exercise a high priority in your life. I make the case for physical activity and explain that regular exercise fundamentally changes your physiology and that this has a profoundly positive affect on your health. To do this, I have compiled ten key benefit groups because there are just too many benefits from exercise to go through them one by one.

In **Chapter 8**, I answer a very important question which you really need to understand: How Long Should You Spend Exercising? I explain the difference between how long and how much and I introduce you to a more objective way to compare different types of exercise done at different levels of intensity. Finally, I introduce you to the Exercise B.A.S.I.C.S. Formula and my 5 Progressive Levels of Exercise, where there is a realistic starting point to suit everyone regardless of your age, weight or current fitness level.

In **Chapter 9**, I answer a second important and related question which you also need to understand: What Type of Exercise Should You Do? I explain the acronym B.A.S.I.C.S., which is easy to understand and remember and the other important part of my Exercise B.A.S.I.C.S. Formula.

In **Chapter 10**, I pull the information from Chapters 8 and 9 together and answer the ultimate question: How should you allocate your exercise time between each kind of exercise? I also introduce you to my training program, the 5X Fitness Transformation, or 5XFT for short.

CHAPTER 6

THIRTEEN OBSTACLES TO EXERCISE

You can find many reasons for not exercising if you are looking for them. Unfortunately, there is far too much inaccurate, or at least misleading, information out there which makes it more difficult than it should be to make the right decisions about exercise. There is very little evidence that exercise is bad for you but there is overwhelming evidence that inactivity is very bad indeed. Inactivity results in such serious health problems as heart disease, stroke, Type 2 Diabetes or even Alzheimer's disease.

There is an emerging theory that too much exercise is unhealthy, but that is referring to extreme endurance activity, which the vast majority of people reading this book do not need to worry about. Bad advice about exercise may cause a host of problems and may also have a negative effect on your ability to exercise in the future. However, the solution to this problem is not to stop exercising, but rather to correct what you are doing wrong and, if necessary, to find alternative forms of exercise.

You already know that there are many people who don't exercise enough; in fact, many do not exercise at all, and there are numerous reasons why. However, I'm sure the main reason is not because they see exercise as harmful, like smoking for instance. So why do people choose not to exercise, especially when they probably know, at least deep down, that they should? I have identified thirteen reasons or obstacles why folks don't exercise, which I will go through one by one.

Your personal circumstances may be such that you are unable to exercise and if that is the case then I sincerely sympathize with you and I hope it is only a temporary situation. However, I think it is more likely that many of you feel that you are unable to exercise because of one or more of these thirteen obstacles. Because exercise is so important to your future, I believe that you have to find a way to overcome these obstacles and in many respects that is why I wrote this book. I hope my comments will help you overcome what is stopping you from exercising.

Obstacle 1—Too Busy

If you feel you are too busy and don't have enough time for exercise, then your problem is probably a priority issue and possibly a time management one, too. If exercise is a low priority in your life, it will always be shoved to the end of the line with your other low priorities and it should be easy to understand why you don't exercise enough.

The solution is therefore clear—you have to change your priorities and place exercise at the top of the list, or at least close to it. In most cases, this will solve the problem because when exercise is a high priority, the "too busy" obstacle seems to fade away. Of course, turning exercise into a high priority when it is currently a low one is far easier said than done, but when you know and understand that it *needs* to be a high priority, it becomes easier to achieve. Much of this book is about persuading you to see exercise as a high priority for the rest of your life. If you are reading this right now you must be at least considering the idea.

If exercise is already a high priority but you are still having problems because you are "too busy", then it is likely that you need to introduce some effective time management techniques, especially regarding exercise. You should definitely plan your exercise time; a helpful technique is to make "exercise appointments" in your diary at the start of each month, or at least at the start of each week, in order to try and build more of a routine into your life. For example, after bringing the kids to school, go to your local gym for spinning or aerobics classes on Tuesday and Thursday mornings. Pay for the classes in advance and commit to do them with a friend. You are much more likely to do them if you make a commitment. And remember—we all get the same twenty-four hours each day and one hundred sixty-eight hours each week!

Obstacle 2—Too Old

This is another common reason why people don't exercise, and I hear it all the time. I believe it is influenced by the tendency for many adults to "retire" from planned exercise in their thirties. We discussed this issue in Chapter 3.

If you feel you are too old for exercise, you will have to change your mindset. *You are not too old and it is never too late to start exercising!* While many older folks choose to be physically inactive, you don't have to be just because they are. There are many, many examples of older people who exercise regularly and who are in great physical condition. You can, too, and I hope by the time you have finished this book you will have changed your mind about exercise.

No exercise, or a lack of it, will actually accelerate the aging process and you will get older quicker! In a sense, it becomes a self-fulfilling prophecy. On the other hand, if you increase your exercise, you will significantly slow down the aging process and you will feel better and younger. Consider this great exercise motto by Dr. Kenneth Cooper, the father of aerobic exercise:

> *"We do not stop exercising because we grow old;*
> *we grow old because we stop exercising."*

Obstacle 3—Too Heavy

If you feel you are too heavy for exercise you *really* need to change your thinking! I know that starting to exercise is hard even under the best of circumstances, and when you are overweight it is harder still. However, you have to draw a line in the sand and start exercising today!

You already know that a lack of exercise has contributed to your weight problems and this will continue until you *make that decision to change*. You need to start believing that you can achieve results if you put your mind to it.

Exercise will change everything for you. Initially, your focus should be on getting into the habit of exercising regularly, working your way up to the recommended minimum weekly level of 3 hours. You need to take it one step at a time and not be disheartened if you don't see immediate results. This is not a quick fix; this is a major lifestyle change!

Look to what others have achieved for inspiration. At a national level, look at what the participants in the *Biggest Loser* TV show have achieved and think about how difficult it was for them at the start. In my local area, participants in the Healthy Charleston Challenge have achieved similar results.

You can do this, too! It all starts with your attitude. This book will help you get started; you will achieve the results you desire and deserve. Once you change your mindset and start to think positively you *will* succeed.

Obstacle 4—Too Tired

If you feel you are too tired, you need to realize that it is the lack of exercise which is making you feel this way. This is counterintuitive, I know, but fatigue is often one of the results of insufficient exercise. Nevertheless, you probably assume that starting to exercise will make you feel even worse. This is usually not the case but you will need just a little faith.

Start exercising and you will see amazing changes over time. You need to be a little patient right at the start because it takes time to reacclimatize your body to exercise. With a little endurance, however, you will achieve this quickly—in fact, you won't even know yourself before too long! You will have a lot more energy, you will not feel as tired, you will sleep a lot better and you will be able to gradually increase the amount of exercise that you do. This will further enhance how you feel and you will begin to see an abundance of benefits as a result.

Obstacle 5—Injured

If you are injured, then of course you need to be careful with your recovery; hopefully it is only a temporary situation. Whenever possible, don't let your injury stop you from exercising, unless you are seriously incapacitated. Talk to your doctor about your injury and rehabilitation, and discuss alternative forms of exercise while you are recuperating.

Guess what? Your recovery program from an injury nearly always includes EXERCISE! You will often get a series of strength building and stretching exercises to do as part of your rehabilitation. However, it is truly important that you don't neglect the uninjured parts of your body during this period.

There is a rule of thumb which states that for every one week you cannot or do not exercise, it will take two weeks to get back to the level of fitness at which you were before you got injured. Keep this in mind, also, and have patience as you work through your recovery.

There are nearly always other forms of exercise that you can do as you recover. For example, when I have been injured in the past, I've done swimming and then some aqua jogging in the same pool. Depending on the injury and the weather, I have often done cycling or spinning as well.

Professional athletes always include exercise as part of their recovery; you should too. You will recover faster and you will benefit from the cross-training. You may even find a new form of exercise you enjoy, that you will want to continue into the future!

Obstacle 6—Arthritis

If you suffer from arthritis, you will probably need to get medical advice. For the majority of you, however, you need to change your thinking. I am a firm believer that exercise helps—it does not hinder—arthritis.

I have bad osteoarthritis in both my big toes and arthritis developing in my knees. Nevertheless, my attitude is that it will get even worse if I stop exercising, so I am not quitting any time soon. When I miss even one day of exercise, my joints will stiffen up and they can be quite sore the next day. Thankfully, though, after about 5 minutes (trust me on this one), they are fine. Now "fine" is a relative term. I can still feel my stiff toes if I think about them—they are a little sore, but not too bad. If they get worse, I usually stop and call it a day!

One last thing. I seldom, if ever, take medication for my arthritis. Occasionally, I may take anti-inflammatories but the pain needs to be very bad. Even then, I only take the medication after I finish exercising. I have taken pain killers before a race but I hate doing it and I don't see it as part of my future. This is, of course, a personal choice but I thought you would like to know my views.

So the bottom line here is that if you do not exercise, your arthritis will get worse; if you exercise, at worst you will slow down the progression of your arthritis—it may even improve. Believe!

Obstacle 7—Doctor

If your doctor says you cannot exercise, then depending on your circumstances, it may be worth seeking a second opinion. In my experience, most (but not all) doctors are sensitive to the benefits of exercise.

I have had my share of doctors tell me that I should stop running because of my arthritis but I'm a big boy and can make up my own mind; so can you! Since my father died from coronary heart disease when I was twenty years old, I have always taken the view that my heart was much more important than my big toes!

I think it is highly unlikely that you will be told to stop exercising altogether; no doctor is going to do this. They may tell you not to ski or not to run but there are many alternatives. Inactivity will lead to a whole host of much greater negative consequences; on the other hand, continuing to exercise and/or finding an alternative form of exercise will be crucial to your long term health.

Obstacle 8—No Good

You may feel you are "no good" at sports. That may be true, but it is not a valid reason for not exercising; it is an excuse. You don't need any talent to walk, run, ride or spin so you have many alternatives to choose from. Yes, there are some things that require skill or talent—like tennis or ballroom dancing—but I am pleased to report from my personal knowledge and experience that this is not the case when it comes to running or riding your bike. As you know, I learned to swim when I was a kid. Why do you think I was able to do triathlons? No talent required!

If you decide to stay inactive because you are "no good" at exercise, then that is your decision, but you should anticipate many future negative consequences. On the other hand, if you take the bull by the horns and make the decision to exercise where no talent is required, you will not regret it!

Obstacle 9—Hate Sports

If you are one of those people who say that you hate all sports and anything to do with exercise, I just don't believe you; that is nothing more than another excuse. Get over it and find something that you like, even if you only like it a little!

If you feel exercise is boring, then find something that you consider a little less boring, such as parasailing or Zumba. Just as I explained in the last reason, if you decide not to exercise you should anticipate many future negative consequences. On the other hand, if you give it a try, you may find that exercise isn't so bad, and I can promise that you will not regret it!

Obstacle 10—Hard Work

If you feel exercise is too much hard work, then consider the time, effort, pain and cost associated with your future poor health. That may be enough to cause you to change your mind! Yes, you have to work at it and yes, it takes some time. Think of it, though, as an investment in your "Health Bank" which will help fight off the potential adverse effects of aging and, in doing so, increase your life expectancy and the quality of your time.

Obstacle 11—Sweaty and Smelly

If you feel you get all sweaty and smelly, then join the club! Welcome to the real world of exercise. Yes, you will get sweaty and even smelly from time to time, though you can sometimes avoid that. Sweating is a sign of being healthy; through perspiration your body is able to eliminate toxins. Think of all the benefits of exercise (see next chapter) and if you still cannot handle the thought of facing your new friends, who, by the way, will all be sweaty and maybe even smelly, too, then you can always do your exercise at home. Remember that you can slip into the changing room or bathroom and change into fresh clothes before joining your friends for coffee!

Obstacle 12—Embarrassed

If you get embarrassed when you exercise, maybe because you feel people are looking at you, then realize this—unless you are beautiful to look at, they are not looking at you. And if you are beautiful, then lucky you!

If you are overweight, I can understand why you might be embarrassed, but remember that there are many people in the same boat. You will get over it as you get used to exercising and especially as you start to lose weight.

Think about all the positive benefits that will emerge once you get started. Also, can I let you in on a little secret? The vast majority of people are on your side and will both support and admire you for your efforts. The few that aren't are not worth worrying about!

Obstacle 13—Expensive

If you feel exercise is too expensive, wait until you see the cost of medical care associated with all the health problems caused by inactivity! There is no doubt that there is a direct cost associated with exercise but it doesn't have to be significant and there are many things you can do to keep your costs down. You do not have to join a gym and you do not have to hire a personal trainer or coach.

Make sure you have a good pair of shoes if you are walking or running. In my view, this is your most important piece of equipment—a "need to have" versus a "nice to have"! If you can, invest in whatever exercise equipment you need. You will find that you will be motivated to wear your new shoes, new outfit, new sunglasses or whatever, and you will be more likely to exercise as a result. This will help you get into the habit of exercising and you will find that the benefits of exercise *significantly* outweigh the costs of inactivity in the long run.

Are You In Control?

You are ultimately in control of your destiny and your future journey. Changing your lifestyle, changing your eating habits and starting to exercise are all within your sphere of control. What you do is your choice and ultimately only you can choose. Sure, you can ask family, friends, colleagues or coaches for advice but ultimately this is your decision.

You must take responsibility for your decisions and stop letting others control your life. You cannot control the world around you, nor can you control the lives of other people. You can, however, control the choices that *you* make in *your* life. Who is driving your life? Are you in the driver's seat or are you just a passenger? Make your decision today to get in the driver's seat, take responsibility for your own choices and get where you need to go; this is a much more rewarding way to live your life.

Sometimes you have to take a leap of faith. Believe in yourself and dive right in; there is light at the end of the tunnel! Take that next step and maximize the quality of your life! You are responsible for the decisions you make in your life, the good ones as well as the bad. You must take control of your life and once you do, there is no going back. The only person stopping you is you!

Some Final Thoughts

While there are many obstacles to exercise, there are just as many solutions and if you want to, you can decide to find them! There is an illustration I want to make by referring to the hit TV show, *The Biggest Loser*. Those of you who have watched it will readily identify with what I am about to say. If you have not watched it, then I ask you to try to visualize the scenario I am about to describe.

Think about the participants in the final weeks of the competition. They are all totally motivated, without exception. Those remaining in the competition talk about winning it, not just about losing weight, and those who have gone home are still working hard to achieve their personal goals. Collectively, their achievements are amazing, which is a huge credit to both them and the show. They are completely and utterly transformed—no longer are they the same participants who started the competition a few months earlier. Do you remember them falling off treadmills, puking their guts up, crying and sometimes even coming close to throwing in the towel?

While your experience does not need to be as "brutal" as the *Biggest Loser*, it will be tough—very tough!—at the start. Accordingly, you need to prepare yourself for a challenge that will be great, but will be well worth facing. By the way, this phenomenon applies to most new things that you start!

So, if you decide to start exercising, and I really hope you do, remember that starting is usually the hardest part. However, if you persevere and refuse to give up, you will come through this successfully and get the results you deserve. Make sure you start slowly and progress gradually to avoid the kind of excessive pain experienced by the *Biggest Loser* participants; this is very important.

In conclusion, there are many, sometimes self-imposed, reasons for not exercising which you can overcome. In my opinion, though, the many benefits of exercise greatly outweigh the costs associated with it, as you will see in the next chapter.

✗ Your "To Do" List

Because taking control of your life and overcoming these obstacles is so important, my to do list in this chapter provides actions you can take to help you overcome whatever is stopping you from exercising. There is one action for each of the thirteen obstacles.

1. Exercise must become a high priority in your life. When it does, it becomes a whole lot easier to find the time required and you will benefit accordingly.
2. You have to change your mindset about exercise in order to decelerate the aging process. Remember—we don't stop exercising because we grow old; we grow old because we stop exercising.
3. You must believe that you *can* exercise and that you *will* lose weight. Believing you can lose weight will help you exercise and exercise will help you lose weight.
4. Just start exercising. As your energy increases you will be able to do more and you will benefit greatly.
5. If you are injured, you need time to recover, but don't stop exercising! Find another form of exercise and you will recover faster and benefit long term.
6. You must at least test my belief that exercise will help your arthritis, whereas inactivity will exacerbate it.
7. Make sure your doctor supports whatever exercise is appropriate for you. If he does not, it would be worth your while to at least seek a second opinion.
8. Don't say you are no good at exercise. You don't need talent for most activities. Make the decision to exercise and you will not regret it.
9. There has to be at least one form of exercise you like. Find it!
10. Change your mindset about exercise. Yes, it is hard work, especially at the start, but you will find that, like most things worth fighting for, it is absolutely worth it.

11. Yes, you will sweat, but remember—the more you sweat, the greater the benefits!

12. Take a leap of faith! Most people will support and admire your efforts to exercise so there is no need to feel embarrassed.

13. Think long term and do the math. There are financial costs to exercise but it is far more expensive if you don't.

"We do not stop exercising because we grow old;
we grow old because we stop exercising."
—Dr. Kenneth Cooper

CHAPTER 7

HOW TO MAKE EXERCISE A HIGH PRIORITY IN YOUR LIFE

T he evidence supporting the case for exercise is as significant as the evidence which demonstrates the dangers of inactivity. These messages go hand-in-hand and they are a critical part of the solution to the very difficult and challenging health problems facing America and the world. Regular exercise fundamentally changes your physiology, including your circulatory, respiratory, musculoskeletal and nervous systems. This has a profoundly positive effect on your health and especially on your ability to lose and maintain weight.

Except in very extreme cases, there are no situations I can think of where no exercise would be better than at least some. Nonetheless, to benefit from exercise, it is very important to treat it with the respect it deserves. This is very important if you are older, if you have been inactive for some time or especially if you are significantly overweight. (Body Mass Index 25–29.9 is overweight; 30 and above is considered obese)

Conservative Approach

In my experience, one of the reasons exercise gets a bad rap is because many people start out too aggressively and get injured at an early stage. This can be demoralizing and often leads to folks giving up because they incorrectly assume that exercise just isn't for them. Because it is so important, I want to highlight the need to be conservative, especially when starting out. To get the maximum benefit from exercise, *you should always start your exercise program slowly with small, gradual steps toward your goal.* More often than not, the hare will lose to the tortoise!

Ten Key Benefit Groups

There are just too many benefits from exercise to go through them one by one; that would be a book all by itself! So I have put them all into ten key groups or categories as follows:

Group 1—Overall Health Benefits

There are so many health benefits associated with exercise that it has to be at the top of my list. Regular exercise plays a critical role in your overall health and it significantly lowers the risk of heart disease, stroke, cancer, diabetes, stress, sleep disorders and depression. It also increases longevity and lowers the risks associated with aging, including Alzheimer's, other forms of dementia, arthritis and osteoporosis.

Group 2—Everyone Benefits

Regular exercise provides health and many other benefits for everyone! Every age group, from children and adolescents to young and middle-aged adults to older adults, benefits. People in every studied ethnic group, including those with disabilities, benefit from exercise.

Group 3—More Is Better

There is no consensus among fitness experts on this issue, increasing the likelihood of confusion among people. I believe that in most cases more exercise is better and *some* exercise is always better than none. Additional benefits occur as the amount of exercise increases, both in greater frequency and longer duration.

There are many different types of exercise and we will explore this further in Chapter 9. Aerobic exercise or cardio, muscle strengthening (resistance), stretching and higher intensity activities are all very beneficial. The benefits from most forms of exercise far outweigh the possibility of adverse outcomes.

Group 4—Healthy Muscles and Bones

I mentioned earlier that regular exercise fundamentally changes many aspects of your physiology. This is especially true of your musculoskeletal system. Regular exercise improves your posture, balance and coordination and it will slow down sarcopenia, the gradual loss of muscle mass which starts at about age thirty. This continues at the rate of between 0.5% and 1% a year and accelerates in your late fifties and early sixties.

It doesn't have to be like this; by exercising regularly and especially by including muscle strengthening in your exercise program, you can significantly postpone this process. You will also improve joint function and strengthen your bones which will increase your pain resistance and reduce the risk of arthritis and osteoporosis.

Group 5—Healthy Heart

This one is so important that it deserves a group all on its own. Your heart is possibly the most important beneficiary of all; it profits from exercise from the moment it starts beating right to your very last beat. Exercise makes your heart stronger and has a profoundly positive effect on your blood circulation, including blood pressure, cholesterol levels and oxygen supply to your cells.

So think about this just for a moment: if your heart benefits from exercise right up until the moment you die, why would you ever want to stop? Why would you even consider giving up something which is so beneficial for your heart, especially when inactivity makes everything so much worse?

Group 6—Healthy Brain

While your heart is one key beneficiary from exercise, so is your brain. As I find it hard to choose between my brain and my heart, I am going to take the easy option and call it a tie. Seriously, you should think about the wellbeing of your brain (using it to do so) as much as your heart—especially as you get older.

Exercise is critically important to your brain's health and it protects against aging and dementia, including Alzheimer's disease. It keeps your brain fit and boosts mental health; it sharpens your concentration and memory and improves learning ability. It also boosts creative thinking and makes you feel happier. So just like your heart, why would you ever even think about hurting this critical organ you use every day of your life by giving up exercise? A healthy brain is so important that I have devoted Chapter 18, Mind Your Brain, to this subject.

Group 7 — Stress Control

Closely linked to your brain, exercise will have a very positive affect on how you feel. It will lift your mood and reduce stress, which in turn will reduce feelings of anxiety and depression. Exercise will also improve your sleep patterns.

I know from my own personal experience that exercise does relieve stress. Whenever I feel stressed out, I know that if I exercise I will feel much better afterwards. It doesn't really matter what I do, though for me running is my go-to activity in these situations. These runs are usually alone, giving me time to think and make the decisions I need to make, which helps to reduce the stress.

What is going on here? Exercise, especially that done at moderate intensity (like a slow run), causes neurochemicals such as endorphins and dopamine to be released into the brain. This can result in mood changes and the famed "runner's high". Give it a try; there is a strong chance it will work for you, too!

Group 8 — Increased Energy and Endurance

Exercise gives you more energy and reduces fatigue; it sounds counterintuitive but it's true! Regular exercise increases your endurance and makes you fitter and stronger, which means you will have more energy all the time. This, in turn, will also boost your immune system and help prevent colds.

The more energy and endurance you have the more focus you will have and the more productive you will be. If you are concerned about sports, the fitter you are the better your sports performance will be. This always reminds me of my time helping the Mount Pleasant Track Club, the biggest and best youth track and cross-country team in South Carolina. Our kids were always much fitter and faster than kids training for other sports such as baseball, football, soccer and basketball. Many other coaches didn't seem to understand that the fitness level of their kids was a major component of their team's success.

Group 9 — Weight Control

Every health expert on the planet agrees that exercise is an essential ingredient in effective weight loss and control. It will help to improve your eating habits and it reduces the risk of both diabetes and pre-diabetes. Exercise will give you greater confidence and help you build self-esteem. It will also help you to improve your body image and control addictions.

Exercise "turbo-charges" your efforts to lose and control your weight. It is so important to your body's overall health that you are better off being a little overweight and exercising regularly than being a normal weight but not exercising at all. Of course best of all is to exercise regularly and in time reach and maintain a normal weight.

Group 10 — Better Metabolism

There is no doubt that regular exercise improves your metabolism, which allows you to burn calories (including stored fat) more efficiently. This is a major benefit when you are trying to lose or maintain your weight. Higher intensity exercise and muscle strengthening will improve your metabolism even further but you need to take great care here as you can only do so much of this.

In addition, since muscle is metabolically about three times more active at rest than fat, the more you can slow down the loss of muscle mass (sarcopenia), as mentioned in number four above, the better. Each pound of muscle burns approximately six calories a day compared to two calories a day for fat.

Exercise—A High Priority in Your Life

Hopefully by now, if you weren't already, you are convinced of the many benefits of exercise. Regular exercise should be a high priority in your life. Ideally, exercise needs to be such a fundamental part of your life that you look forward to it each day and enjoy it as a natural form of fun and entertainment. I believe that if we could truly embrace exercise in this way and make it part of our daily lifestyles, as we often do for our kids, we would solve the inactivity epidemic and all the related health problems much faster than we are likely to do otherwise. Consequently, I am going to continue my analysis of the benefits of exercise by making the case for this important principle.

Exercise must not be considered a chore. I have already referred to the fact that in many circles exercise is presented as a time-consuming "pain in the neck", which you should try to complete and get out of the way as quickly as possible. An increasing number of "fitness experts" are promoting the "less is more" view of exercise; their approach is that you only need to do, say, fifteen to twenty minutes of high intensity exercise, three times a week. As a result, they commonly say that spending any more time than this, especially on lower intensity exercise, is a complete waste of time.

In my view, not only is this advice incorrect but it is potentially dangerous for many people, including older folks in their forties and above—especially those who have been inactive for a long time. It also misses the most important point of all.

Most Valuable Time of the Day

I fully understand and agree that your time is very valuable and because it is, you should spend your time efficiently. However, exercise is not something you should do just because it is good for you, like eating spinach or broccoli. It should not be something that you try to get out of the way as quickly as possible so that you can check it off your list. The fact is that the time I spend exercising is my most special and valuable time of the day and yours should be too. I wouldn't trade it or give it away for anything and you couldn't pay me enough to make me give up my exercise time.

I hope that exercise is a high priority in your life, but just because I think exercise is great doesn't mean you will, too. So I have identified five easy steps that will help you make exercise a high priority in and a fundamental part of your life. Besides all the health benefits mentioned above, you will achieve great results simply by taking these actions. You can make exercise more enjoyable, more entertaining and more fun, not just for yourself but for your family, too. Let's go through each one in turn as follows:

Step 1—Make it Fun and Enjoyable!

Exercise should always be a fun and enjoyable time of your day. This is a critical idea to understand and believe. If you see exercise as a waste of time—a chore you are only doing because you feel you have to—then it is time to change your mindset. The best way to do that is to give fun a try! You have to give it a serious chance to succeed and this means trying it a number of times. Exercise is a very positive experience for me and it is my hope and wish that you will see it and experience it the same way. There are many things that you can do to make your exercise more enjoyable and fun. Everyone is different but here are a few of the things I like doing:

- Running is my favorite exercise and I can do this almost anywhere; there is nothing better than to get up early on a Saturday or Sunday morning and run with my family and friends.
- Just going out for a long walk at any time can be a great way to unwind and leave your worries behind for an hour or two. Or, go for an easy bike ride in your neighborhood with your family.
- Cycling trips are great fun. My own favorite place is the Cork and Kerry mountains in the southwest corner of Ireland, referred to by Thin Lizzy in their signature tune "Whiskey in the Jar".
- In the winter, I love to go skiing. This is not only great exercise but also a fun and enjoyable time. I realize skiing can be expensive and takes some organization but once you start you will never want to stop.
- Swimming in the sea can be exhilarating—so much better than a pool! If you try this, make sure you know the terrain and always swim parallel to the shore, preferably in shallow water.

So make a change in your mindset about exercise! Give some of these suggestions a try and you just might find that exercise not only provides health and fitness benefits but it can be a lot of fun, too!

Step 2—Build Relationships

Exercise provides you with a great opportunity to spend more time with your spouse, your kids, your extended family and friends—how great is that! This quality time gives you the opportunity not only to develop great relationships with the most important people in your life, but to do so in a very healthy environment! I have some friends that I've only ever met in the evening for dinner, which, when you think about it, is not such a great idea!

Exercise is also a great way to develop new relationships and friends. Our Saturday and Sunday morning runs have enabled Maureen and me to make some great new friends. We often go for breakfast afterwards, which is also great fun. We would never have developed these new friendships without exercise. The bottom line is this—you should use exercise to develop existing relationships and make new ones; either way, you will achieve better results from both the exercise and the relationships.

Step 3—Cultivate Personal Time

While I like to spend time exercising with my family and friends, I also like to exercise alone and when I can, I split my time between both. Exercise gives you a great window of time for some personal space to unwind from all the stress and pressure in your life. It gives you time and solitude to contemplate and meditate; this is very important. It is also a great way to spend time thinking about things—you will be amazed at how creative you can be! Most of my best ideas occur when I am exercising; in fact, my family will tell you that the first thing I do when I get back home from a run is to go straight into my office and write my ideas down before I forget them.

I regularly spend time mentally preparing for meetings and rehearsing speeches when I exercise alone. And don't underestimate the constructive "time out" that exercise gives you to cool down after an argument! It allows me to calm down, reflect and resolve disputes. So use some of your exercise time as essential personal reflection time and you will be more effective in your life, while getting all the benefits of exercise at the same time.

Step 4—Enjoy the Outdoors

You may have noticed that all the exercise examples I listed in Step 1 above were outdoors. For me, exercising indoors is a last resort. Recently, I was at a conference in Las Vegas and while the few that exercised went to the hotel fitness center, I was out running on the Strip; who do you think had more fun and entertainment? I met a guy named Mike on the way and we ended up running together for about twenty minutes, comparing stories from our weekend.

Try to exercise outdoors every chance you get. You will get to know and enjoy your local environment and I promise you will not regret it. I can think of many great locations to enjoy exercise in Mt. Pleasant, SC where I live but my favorite is my local beach—the Isle of Palms. I am fortunate enough to be able to run there every other weekend, when the tide is out, and it is great for both the mind and the soul.

I realize that bad weather can be a limiting factor but it doesn't have to be. Keep an eye on the weather and work your exercise around it; call your exercise partner and go an hour earlier or later. Change the time you exercise according to the time of year. It gets hot in South Carolina during the summer so I exercise early in the morning. When it is cold, I exercise in the afternoon, which is the warmest part of the day; I am getting soft in my old age!

So try exercising outdoors and you will open up a whole new world and see how your time exercising is both more enjoyable and effective.

Step 5—Benefit from Trips and Vacations

I always make exercise the focus of my vacations; in fact, I cannot remember the last trip I made when I didn't exercise. I always pack my sneakers but those of you who know me will probably say that I am always wearing them, which is true!

Over the years, I have had my fair share of ski and bike trips and fitness-oriented vacations. As a family, we will always choose active vacations where we can do lots of exercise, including running, swimming, cycling, water skiing, snorkeling, etc. I have often built vacations around the completion of marathons and triathlons.

So planned exercise should also be an important element of your trips and vacations. Make sure you pack your gear when you travel so you can maintain your exercise routine wherever you go. Exercising is a great way to explore new places whether you are walking, running, cycling, skiing, rowing or all of the above.

Conclusion

In a nutshell, seeing exercise as a chore and trying to get it out of the way quickly is not very smart at all. Reducing your exercise to about an hour a week, even if it is three short fifteen- or twenty-minute high intensity sessions, just won't cut it.

I believe I have made a strong case for you to make exercise a positive force in your life and to treat it as the high priority it needs to be. If you do this, it will become a fundamental part of your new lifestyle.

✗ Your "To Do" List

1. Start your exercise program slowly with small, gradual steps to achieve the maximum benefit in the longer term.
2. Familiarize yourself with each of the ten benefit groups above; this knowledge will motivate you to exercise.
3. Follow the five steps to make your exercise fun and it will become an important part of your life.
4. Decide today to make exercise a high priority for the rest of your life.

"So many people spend their health gaining wealth
and then have to spend their wealth to regain their health."
—A.J. Reb Materi

CHAPTER 8

HOW LONG SHOULD YOU
SPEND EXERCISING?

You will recall my hypothesis from Chapter 2 that the vast majority of Americans do not exercise enough. To validate my hypothesis, I asked the important question:

How much is enough exercise?

To help me answer the question, I referred to the 2008 *Physical Activity Guidelines for Americans*, reinforced by the World Health Organization and a major research study. My conclusions were as follows:

- **3 hours a week is the minimum recommended level of exercise.**
- **7 hours a week is the optimum level.**

Your Current Fitness Level

The primary objective of any exercise program should be *to sustain and improve your fitness and health on an ongoing basis*. Therefore, you need to take your current level of fitness (see Chapter 13) into account before you decide how long you should spend exercising or how much exercise you should do. If you are currently inactive or you exercise less than the minimum recommended amount of three hours, then you need to gradually work your way up to the minimum level before you progress beyond that point.

If you try to do too much too quickly, you greatly increase your risk of injury. If you get injured you will have to stop before you really get started! I see this happen all the time. Perhaps even more importantly, if your exercise is too hard, you will not enjoy it and it will be more difficult to sustain your motivation in the long-term. I want you to have fun and enjoy your exercise from this day forward!

Follow this advice and you will be able to achieve your fitness goals and maximize your health benefits. At each stage of your progression you should know how much time you need to spend exercising overall, as well as how you should allocate that time to each type of exercise.

How Long Versus How Much

There is an important difference between these questions:

1. How *long* should you spend exercising?
2. How *much* exercise should you do? (or How much exercise is enough?)

How long you spend exercising simply measures time. While it is an important measure, it provides no information about the quality or intensity of your exercise. How much is enough or how much exercise you should do is a better measure because it takes both the quantity (time) and quality (intensity) of your exercise into account.

The Exercise B.A.S.I.C.S. Formula

You may have heard of my Exercise B.A.S.I.C.S. Formula and you may have seen my videos series. If not, you will find them at **www.GetAmericaMoving.com/basics/**.

The Exercise B.A.S.I.C.S. Formula answers two very important questions:

1. **How long should you spend exercising?**
2. **What type of exercise should you do?**

The two questions are closely related to each other because you really need to know what type of exercise you should do before we can completely or comprehensively answer how long you should spend doing it.

I will answer the first question—how long you should spend exercising—in this chapter. I will also introduce you to an easy way to measure how much exercise you do so that you can distinguish between quantity and quality. In the next chapter, I will answer the second question—what type of exercise you should do—and then I will pull it all together by explaining how you should allocate your total exercise time to each type of exercise.

Exercise Intensity

As mentioned above, the question about how much exercise you should do has a qualitative dimension as well as a quantitative one. This qualitative aspect is an important variable we need to consider; that is, the dimension of exercise intensity.

The 2008 *Physical Activity Guidelines* focus on two levels of intensity, which are described as "moderate" and "vigorous". What exactly, though, is moderate intensity and what is vigorous intensity? Are there more than two levels of exercise intensity? Could my vigorous be the same as your moderate intensity or vice versa? By themselves, moderate and vigorous are subjective terms.

The *Guidelines* describe moderate exercise as working hard enough to raise your heart rate and to break a sweat, while vigorous exercise is breathing heavily and raising your heart rate quite a bit. They say that while doing moderate exercise you should be able to talk, but not sing. However, you shouldn't be able to say more than a few words without pausing for breath while doing vigorous exercise.

The *Guidelines* also describe a brisk walk as moderate exercise and "jogging" as vigorous exercise. While this may be correct if you have been inactive or if you don't exercise very much, it is not accurate if you are relatively fit. There is a rule of thumb for runners which says that when you reach the point where you can hold a conversation with your running partners for thirty minutes, you have arrived as a runner. Yet this would be considered easy running (my definition of jogging) and certainly not vigorous. So you can see the problem in using subjective terms like "moderate" and "vigorous" to describe exercise intensity.

Say Hello to the MET

There is a more objective way for us to describe exercise intensity. A common measure used by researchers for this purpose is called the MET. It refers to the amount of energy used by exercising for a fixed period of time—an hour, for example. It sounds technical, especially when its full name is used (Metabolic Equivalent Task), but I promise that will be the first and last time I will use it. Let's simply refer to this measure as the MET, because it is a helpful convention which allows us to compare the relative intensity of different physical activities.

A MET is the ratio of the rate of energy used during a physical activity versus the rate of energy expended at rest for the average person. I have produced **METS Table 1** below to demonstrate the relative intensities of popular physical activities. You can see that the amount of energy used at rest (1 MET) is the basis to which everything else is compared. Please take a minute to study this table.

METS Table 1

Energy Used for Popular Physical Activities	METS
Energy Used At Rest	1.0
Slow Walking—2 miles per hour	2.8
Moderate Walking—3 miles per hour	3.3
Calisthenics (easy exercises)	3.3
Cycling—less than 10 miles per hour	4.0
Fast Walking—4 miles per hour	5.0
Cycling—10 miles per hour	6.0
Slow Running—4.25 miles per hour	6.6

Source: 2011 Compendium of Physical Activities

Not Perfect, but Helpful

The MET is not a perfect measure because it refers to average energy expenditure and thus is not specific to an individual. Actual energy expenditure during exercise depends on a person's body weight; the heavier the body, the greater the energy expenditure. However, it is definitely a helpful measure, especially if you want to understand why it is so important to exercise beyond Levels 1 and 2 of the *Physical Activity Guidelines.*

METS are used to compare the relative intensity of exercise and they can also be expressed in MET Minutes. For example, cycling at ten miles per hour (6 METS) for thirty minutes is equal to energy expenditure of 180 MET Minutes (6 METS x 30 mins.)

Now let's take a look at the exercise options referred to in both Level 1 and Level 2 of the *Physical Activity Guidelines* to illustrate.

Illustration—Level 1 from Physical Activity Guidelines

Option 1

- 150 minutes of "moderate" intensity exercise a week
- Walking at 3 miles per hour = 3.3 METS from Table 1
- Multiply 150 minutes by 3.3 METS
- **500 MET Minutes**

Option 2

- 75 minutes of "vigorous" intensity exercise
- Slow running at 4.25 miles per hour = 6.6 METS from Table 1
- Multiply 75 by 6.6 METS
- **500 MET Minutes**

Option 3

- An equivalent combination of "moderate" and "vigorous" exercise
- Take half of moderate walking + half of slow running from Options 1 and 2
- Add 250 + 250 MET Minutes
- **500 MET Minutes**

PLUS (For All 3 Options)
- Muscle strengthening (calisthenics from Table 1) for 15 minutes, 2 days a week
- Multiply 15 by 2 by 3.3 METS (moderate intensity)
- **100 MET Minutes**

So for all 3 Level 1 Options, you get the same level of energy expenditure:
Total Level 1: 500 + 100 = 600 MET Minutes per Week

Illustration—Level 2 from Physical Activity Guidelines

Option 1
- 300 minutes of "moderate" intensity exercise a week
- Walking at 3 miles per hour = 3.3 METS from Table 1
- Multiply 300 minutes by 3.3 METS
- **1000 MET Minutes**

Option 2
- 150 minutes of "vigorous" intensity exercise
- Slow running at 4.25 miles per hour = 6.6 METS from Table 1
- Multiply 150 minutes by 6.6 METS
- **1000 MET Minutes**

Option 3
- An equivalent combination of "moderate" and "vigorous" exercise
- Take half of moderate walking + half of slow running from Options 1 and 2 above
- Add 500 + 500 MET Minutes
- **1000 MET Minutes**

PLUS (For all 3 options)
- Muscle strengthening (calisthenics from Table 1) for 15 minutes, 2 days a week

- Multiply 15 x 2 x 6.6 METS (vigorous intensity)
- **200 MET Minutes**

So again for all three options for Level 2, you get the same level of energy expenditure:

Total Level 2: 1000 + 200 = 1200 MET Minutes per Week

In both illustrations above, the MET allows us to measure how much exercise is done per week. There are two key variables involved— the amount of time you spend exercising and the intensity of your exercise, which is often measured by your speed (miles per hour) or pace (minutes per mile). The big advantage of using the MET to compare physical activities is that it takes both variables into account at the same time. So let's go back to the illustrations for Level 1 and 2 of the *Physical Activity Guidelines*.

Level 1 from *Physical Activity Guidelines*

	How Long	How Much	Calculations for How Much
Option 1	180 Mins.	600 MET Mins.	150 x 3.3 + 30 x 3.3
Option 2	105 Mins.	600 MET Mins.	75 x 6.6 + 30 x 3.3
Option 3	142.5 Mins.	600 MET Mins.	75 x 3.3 + 37.5 x 6.6 + 30 x 3.3

Clearly, if we can answer the multi-dimensional question "how much," we get more useful information than the one-dimensional "how long". Option three illustrates this very well. If we ask, "How long did you spend exercising?" the answer is 142.5 minutes. If we ask, "How much exercise did you do?" the answer is 75 minutes of walking at 3 MPH (3.3 METS), 37.5 minutes of slow running at 4.25 MPH (6.6 METS) and 30 minutes of strength exercises (3.3 METS) for a total of 600 MET Minutes.

Level 2 from *Physical Activity Guidelines*

	How Long	How Much	Calculation for How Much
Option 1	330 Mins.	1200 MET Mins.	300 x 3.3 + 30 x 6.6
Option 2	180 Mins.	1200 MET Mins.	180 x 6.6
Option 3	255 Mins	1200 MET Mins.	150 x 3.3 + 105 x 6.6

Option three again illustrates the advantage of asking, "How much exercise?" The answer to how long is 255 minutes, whereas the answer to how much is 150 minutes of walking at 3 MPH (3.3 METS), 75 minutes of slow running at 4.25 MPH (6.6 METS) and 30 minutes of more vigorous strength exercises (6.6 METS) for a total of 1200 MET Minutes.

Using METS to Compare Levels

Before we move on, let us review Level 1 vs. Level 2 of the *Physical Activity Guidelines*.

- Level 1 = 600 MET Minutes Per Week
- Level 2 = 1200 MET Minutes Per Week

So, taking both time and intensity into account, Level 2 uses twice the weekly energy expenditure of Level 1. While the *Guidelines* define intensity using METS, the authors maintain that they are not useful for the general public because the idea of METS is too difficult to understand. I respectfully disagree and think it is a useful and helpful way to explain how much exercise you should do without getting too complicated. This is especially true for readers of this book who need to understand why it is so important to exercise beyond Levels 1 and 2.

5 Progressive Levels of Exercise

We know the *Guidelines* say additional and more extensive health benefits are gained by engaging in physical activity beyond Level 2, with the greatest benefits occurring at seven hours of exercise per week. Level 1 is a good starting point, but it is only a stepping stone on the continuum of physical activity. We can extrapolate our weekly physical activity beyond Levels 1 and 2 to achieve additional and more extensive health benefits. Let's say we add three steps to give us **5 Progressive Levels of Exercise,** with each new level a gradual progression from the previous one, adding 600 MET Minutes of weekly energy expenditure each time, as presented in the following graph:

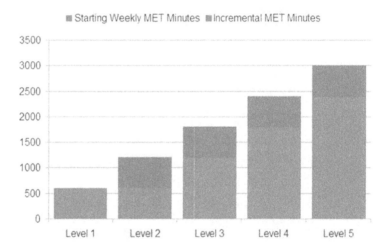

With 5 Progressive Levels of Exercise, there is a realistic starting point to suit everyone and this can be summarized as follows:

Level	Hours of Exercise per Week	Average Days of Exercise per Week	MET Minutes	MET Minutes per Hour
Level 1	3 Hours (Minimum)	4	600	200
Level 2	4 Hours	5	1200	300
Level 3	5 Hours	5	1800	360
Level 4	6 Hours	5	2400	400
Level 5	7 Hours (Optimum)	6	3000	428

The key here is that progression to the next level should always be *gradual*. By doing so, you increase both your time and your intensity, adding 600 MET

Minutes of weekly energy expenditure for each new level. As you increase both your exercise time and intensity, we need to extend our list of physical activities from our earlier METS Table 1.

In METS Table 2 below, I have added columns for miles per hour and minutes per mile to help those of you who like to think this way when exercising. So for example, a fast walking speed of four miles per hour can also be described as a fifteen minute mile pace. The METS value for this pace is five, which is equivalent to 300 MET Minutes per hour (5 METS x 60 mins). Take a few minutes to study METS Table 2; it will be worth it!

METS Table 2

Energy Expended for Popular Exercise	Miles per Hour	Minutes per Mile	METS	MET Minutes
Energy Expended At Rest	0.0	0	1.0	60
Slow Walking—2 miles per hour	2.0	30	2.8	168
Moderate Walking—3 miles per hour	3.0	20	3.3	200
Calisthenics (easy exercises)	0.0	0	3.3	200
Cycling—less than 10 miles per hour	< 10	> 6	4.0	240
Fast Walking—4 miles per hour	4.0	15	5.0	300
Cycling—10 miles per hour	10	6	6.0	360
Slow Running	4.25	14	6.6	400
Calisthenics (vigorous exercises)			7.5	450
Running—5 miles per hour	5.0	12	8.3	498
Running—6 miles per hour	6.0	10	9.8	588
Cycling—15 miles per hour	15	4	10.0	600
Running—8 miles per hour	8.0	7.5	11.8	708

Source: 2011 Compendium of Physical Activities

How Long Should You Spend Exercising?

The answer to the original question asked at the start of this chapter, *"How long should you spend exercising?"* ultimately depends on the results you want to achieve. If you want to:

- live a long and healthy life, free from major illnesses and injuries
- be fit and strong enough to continue doing all the active things you like doing for a long time
- have an active, fun and enjoyable lifestyle in the company of your family and friends
- maintain a healthy weight or lose weight until you get to the level necessary to achieve the above results

then without hesitation, I would strongly recommend, taking into account where you are now, that you gradually work your way up through the 5 Levels. Remember, if you are just starting out, you should start at Level 1 and not move on to Level 2 until you are ready. However, your long-term goal should be to progress to Level 5.

Optimum Level—Seven Hours a Week

The short, simple answer to the above question is that you should gradually work your way up to Level 5—**seven hours a week**, which I believe to be the optimum level of exercise if you want to achieve the health outcomes listed above.

In an ideal world, some exercise every day would be good and so you should try to spread your seven hours out over the week. You should try to do some form of exercise every day, but seven out of seven days is difficult, given our demanding lives. So, if we aim for seven we will have a good chance of actually achieving five or six, which is still very good.

Some days you will feel good and others you will feel bad. That is just the way it is; but as you progress, you will have far more good days than bad days. When you have a bad day, don't worry about it. Just do what you can and come back fighting; tomorrow is another day! On the days that you miss an exercise session, make sure you do as much Baseline exercise as possible.

When you eventually get to Level 5, which you will if you really want to, you may be absolutely content to stay there because this is the optimum exercise level. We really don't know if there are additional benefits beyond this level. When you get there, then you can start thinking about the additional, more advanced steps that will be waiting for you if you are interested. But as the saying goes, let's just take one step (or one level) at a time!

✗ Your "To Do" List

- Establish your current level of fitness (see Chapter 13) and find your correct starting point. Do not try to do too much too quickly.
- Familiarize yourself with the MET and the illustrations and MET tables in this chapter.
- Gradually work your way up through the 5 Progressive Levels of Exercise to the optimum level but do not progress to the next level until you are ready to do so.

*"Everyone is an athlete. The only difference is
that some of us are in training, and some are not."*
—Dr. George Sheehan

Counting Calories

The MET measure is also helpful if you are trying to lose weight as you exercise. That is because we can estimate the number of calories used by applying the following formula:

- Your Weight in Kilograms multiplied by the METS Value of Activity = Calories burned per hour.
- Since 1 Kg = 2.2 lbs, you can convert your weight from pounds to kilograms by dividing by 2.2.
- So, for example, let us assume you are 200 lbs. and you are cycling at 10 miles per hour (6 METS from Table 1) for 1 hour. You calculate calories used as follows:
- 200/2.2 X 6 METS = 545 Calories

Calculating the number of calories used is obviously helpful, especially if you are trying to lose weight. It also pulls together each of the three exercise variables—type of exercise, intensity and time spent—into one number for each workout. If you add your daily calories together you will have the number of calories burned weekly, which you can then compare to 3500—the approximate number of calories required to lose one pound.

It is important to remember that while this is a helpful formula, it is not precise. It is more of an estimate and does not take into account differences in metabolism due to gender, age or body composition, which will all influence the results. There are other formulas out there that you could use instead of this one. Typically, they are more complicated (e.g. American College of Sports Medicine[7]), but they are still all estimates at the end of the day.

---

7   Bushman, B. American College of Sports Medicine. (2014). *Factors The Influence Daily Calorie Needs*. Retrieved from http://www.acsm.org.

CHAPTER 9

WHAT TYPE OF EXERCISE SHOULD YOU DO?

n the last chapter, I explained the important difference between how long you should spend exercising and how much exercise you should do. For your convenience, I have reproduced the key details below.

Weekly Exercise	Level 1 (Minimum)	Level 2	Level 3	Level 4	Level 5 (Optimum)
Days/Week	4	5	5	5	6
Hours/Week	3	4	5	6	7
METS/ Week	600	1200	1800	2400	3000

Now that you know how much exercise you should do in terms of days and hours per week as well as MET minutes per week, you will also want answers to the following questions:

- What type of exercise should you do?
- How should you allocate your time to each type of exercise?

We will answer the first question in this chapter and then we will pull it all together in Chapter 10: How to Allocate Your Exercise Time.

What is Exercise?

As I sat down to write this section, I realized that before I answered the question "What type of exercise should you do?" it would be helpful to define exactly what I mean by the term "exercise". The first things that popped into my mind were: physical activity, fitness and health, in that order. But rather than try to reinvent the wheel by coming up with my own definition, I decided to look it up. I was pleasantly surprised with the following definition from the Oxford Dictionaries:

> *"Exercise is an activity requiring physical effort, carried out especially to sustain or improve health and fitness."*

What I really like about this definition is the emphasis it places on **sustaining and improving** health and fitness because that is what you should always seek to do when you exercise. So it is crucially important that whatever exercise you do, you meet that standard of at least sustaining, but preferably improving, your health and fitness over time.

One problem with the word exercise is that it is such a broad term, which covers a multitude of different physical activities from aerobics classes to Zumba. Moreover, it includes all sports such as football, baseball, soccer, basketball, volleyball and tennis. Oh, and don't forget my favorite sport— rugby! Seven a side rugby, which is an amazing game, will be included in the Olympic Games in Rio De Janeiro for the first time in 2016. The tip rugby I referred to earlier in the book is like sevens, except without all the rough physical stuff. But I digress.

Exercise also includes aerobic activities, often referred to as cardio, such as walking, jogging, running, swimming, biking, rowing, kayaking and skiing. It includes strength training with weight machines and free weights as well as calisthenics and circuit training, which is my favorite. Circuit training is usually done using your own body weight for resistance. Activities such as yoga or Pilates include strength training, stretching and flexibility. Cross-training is a term used to describe exercise covering two or more activities, such as running and swimming. It also includes increasingly popular sports like duathalon (running/cycling) and triathlon (swimming/cycling/running).

So to answer the question "What type of exercise should you do?" I have created an acronym, which is both easy to understand and remember. I call it the B.A.S.I.C.S. and it is a key part of my Exercise B.A.S.I.C.S. Formula, which I referred to earlier.

The B.A.S.I.C.S.

The six letters in the acronym represent the following forms of exercise:

B = Baseline
A = Aerobic
S = Strength
I = Intensity
C = Cross-training
S = Stretching

I describe exercise as the "secret sauce" to a long, high quality life. To achieve this, the B.A.S.I.C.S. implies that for **optimum** fitness and health you should be doing some of each element. When employed together, these components will boost your fitness and health—especially that of your circulatory system, your heart and your brain. They will also boost your metabolism; this means you will burn energy more effectively which, in turn, will help you to lose or control your weight.

Just Starting Out

The type of exercise you should do depends on your current exercise level. If you are just starting out at Level 1, which is the minimum exercise level, your initial focus should be on these four elements of the B.A.S.I.C.S:

Baseline + Aerobic + Strength + Stretching

You should add higher intensity and cross-training as you move gradually through the 5 Progressive Levels of Exercise. I will now explain why as I go through each element of the B.A.S.I.C.S.

B—Baseline

Baseline exercise is a term used to describe all the unplanned activities of normal daily life from the time we get up in the morning to the time we go to sleep at night. It includes all physical activities such as standing, walking, eating, sitting, housework, lifting light objects, etc. While people vary in how much baseline activity they do, those who only do baseline activities (i.e. no planned exercise) are generally considered inactive, which may or may not be fair. For example, it is likely that a farm hand gets a lot more baseline exercise than a typical office worker.

Over the centuries, human beings have made much progress on nearly every front that you care to think of. This is especially true of the last thirty or forty years, where the rate of change has accelerated very rapidly. Unfortunately, a negative byproduct of all this progress and new technology is that we do far less baseline activity today than we have in the past.

I have witnessed these dramatic changes during my lifetime. Let me give you a few examples: your remote control means you do not have to leave your chair when watching TV. Fast food drive-thrus mean you do not have to leave your car to eat breakfast, lunch or dinner. Online shopping means you do not have to leave your home to buy many kinds of products and services, whereas before you had to go out to go shopping. All of this is great progress for humankind but what does it mean for your health and fitness?

This gradual reduction in physical activity, by stealth, has contributed to the health problems we now face and if we let it continue, things will get worse. Consequently, we have to take action to restore the balance and we can start by changing our mindset towards baseline activities. This means ***baseline exercise needs to be a high priority!***

Baseline Activities You Can Do

If you have a positive attitude or mindset, there is a lot you can do to increase your baseline activities every day. While we do not have any direct evidence that more baseline exercise will result in health benefits, there is no question in my mind that it must help and you should do all you can to increase it. At a minimum, it burns calories and it can help you maintain a healthy body weight. So consider adding the following baseline activities to your daily routine:

- Walk or cycle instead of driving whenever you can. Park your car further away from your destination and walk. Next time you go to a fast food restaurant, do not join the drive-thru; park your car away from the door and walk into the restaurant to get your food. Of course, I know you know that too much fast food is not good for you, so try to cut back.

- Take the stairs whenever you can instead of using the elevator in offices, hotels, airports, etc. See how many flights you can climb without getting too winded. If you struggle, you have some clear evidence that you need to increase your fitness level. However, as you get better at this, you will soon be taking two steps at a time and getting a mini workout done.

- A slight twist on the last one is to use your stairs at home as often as possible. Create reasons to take more trips up and down the stairs by dividing things up into smaller, lighter loads. It might seem inefficient, but the additional exercise will help you.

- Increase the amount of walking you do at work during coffee and lunch breaks. If you pick your kids up from the school bus, meet them a stop or two earlier and walk home.

- Drink plenty of water, which is both good for you and will mean more trips to the bathroom. Go to the bathroom farthest away!

- Limit the amount of time you spend watching TV and/or playing computer games, and replace this time with physical activities. Go for a short walk after dinner instead of falling asleep watching TV. It will aid digestion and help you sleep better.

- If you can, stand at home, at work or at play instead of sitting all the time; this simple adjustment will burn up at least twice the amount of energy (calories), which will also help you control your weight. Do this especially when talking on the phone.

A great way to observe your progress with baseline exercise is to track your additional daily movements with a GPS watch or pedometer. Some people find it very motivational to have the evidence before their eyes on a daily basis.

Sitting Has Become the New Smoking

There is a negative correlation between the amount of time you spend sitting every day and your health. The more you sit, the worse your health, and this applies even if your planned exercise is at the optimum level of seven hours a week!

This is a relatively new but very scary development and I certainly didn't hear about it until very recently. I have practiced what I preached for a long time now regarding planned exercise and I am very conscious about what is happening to baseline exercise. However, I am also guilty of sitting for long periods of time. The vast majority of my work is done sitting and so the more and harder I work, the more I endanger myself. I have to admit that I also like to watch television at night and I also watch rugby games at the weekend.

Increasing research suggests that sitting increases your risk of death and disease even if you are getting plenty of exercise. It is just like smoking; it's bad for you regardless of the amount of planned exercise you do every day. Unfortunately, it seems that outside of our planned exercise sessions, active folks, like me, sit just as much, if not more than inactive folks. As mentioned earlier in Part 1, in a study published in the *International Journal of Behavioral Nutrition and Physical Activity* researchers reported that people spent an average of sixty-four hours a week sitting, which is more than nine hours a day, regardless of how active they were.

They were also surprised to learn that many of those doing higher amounts of exercise inadvertently made less effort to exercise outside of their planned exercise time. Further research from Illinois State University reported that people were about 30% less active overall on days when they exercised versus days that they didn't. I can identify with this as you are likely to feel you should rest more on days that you exercise.

I am sure the significance and importance of this development is not lost on you and it really emphasizes the importance of making baseline exercise, as well as planned exercise, a high priority in your life. You need to build the kind of baseline activities suggested above into your daily routine.

A—Aerobic

Aerobic exercise includes physical activities such as walking, jogging, running, swimming, biking, kayaking, rowing, skiing, etc. As a longtime runner and triathlete, I am very definitely a proponent of including aerobic exercise, often referred to as "cardio" or "endurance", in your weekly exercise routine.

Unfortunately, aerobic exercise increasingly gets a bad rap in some quarters and is sometimes described as boring or a waste of time. Some experts say that you are always better off focusing on quality rather than quantity when you exercise. While intuitively this makes sense, with exercise it just doesn't work that way. I believe that there is a lot of confusing and sometimes misleading information out there about cardio, or aerobic, exercise, which I am going to try to clarify in this section.

I have listed below ten reasons why I believe aerobic exercise is very important and must be included as an integral part of your weekly exercise program.

10 Reasons Why You Must Do Aerobic Exercise

1. **Health Benefits:** Aerobic exercise provides many health benefits— especially if you are older, overweight or out of shape. There may be some issues with extreme levels of aerobic activity but the vast majority of people reading this book do not need to worry about this.

2. **Always Better Than None:** Aerobic exercise is always better and hugely more beneficial than no exercise at all; it is certainly not a waste of time! However, there are more effective ways to exercise if all you ever do is aerobic exercise or cardio at the same pace. Even so, exercising at one pace is much easier said than done, and is very difficult for beginners to achieve.

3. **Built-In Intensity:** The reality is that the vast majority of people who do aerobic exercise do not do it at the same pace; for many, including runners, swimmers, bikers, skiers, kayakers, etc. there are built-in increases in intensity (think about hills, the wind, the tide, etc.)

4. **Never Easy at the Start:** This is especially true if you have been inactive and are just starting out. I am sure you can relate to the fact that even "easy" aerobic exercise at the start is not easy! My opinion is that it is best to start slowly and *gradually* build up your volume and intensity so that your confidence grows; you enjoy your exercise more and, perhaps most importantly of all, you avoid injury. Over the years I have seen far too many folks stop exercising because of injuries caused by trying to do too much too quickly.

5. **Every Workout:** In my view, it is always a serious mistake to go from naught to sixty when you are exercising. This is especially true when you are just starting out or trying to get back into aerobic exercise. Serious athletes always warm up, stretch and do stride-outs before doing sprints or high intensity interval training (HIIT). So should you! Thus, every workout you do should include a ten minute warm-up and a ten minute cool down, which is aerobic exercise.

6. **Professionals:** Almost every serious athlete on the planet does aerobic exercise, with very few exceptions. In the past, sprinters and heavy weightlifters may have tried to avoid it, but I would be surprised if many do today. Certainly the more successful ones don't shun aerobic exercise. In fact, for most athletes, aerobic exercise is a fundamental part of their training, especially when they are warming up, cooling down and in recovery mode.

7. **Important Part:** Long distance runners, swimmers, cyclists and triathletes obviously do plenty of aerobic exercise. However, they also do high intensity interval training, strength training and cross-training, as well as stretching and flexibility routines. Your body needs time to recover from your high intensity and strength days and you can do this by resting (no planned exercise at all) or by having a recovery day with easy aerobic exercise. As you progress and gain experience, aerobic exercise will play an increasingly important role in your weekly training.

8. **Fun and Enjoyment:** All exercise, but especially aerobic exercise, should be fun and enjoyable. You should aim to get maximum pleasure and enjoyment from all your exercise and you will find that aerobic exercise provides the greatest opportunity for you to do this!

9. **In The Zone:** As you progress, you can look forward to long, easy aerobic exercise where you are "in the zone", whether you are running, swimming, biking, skiing, kayaking, etc. When you get there, you will experience your aerobic exercise like never before. It is, as it should be, a time of great enjoyment, peace and creativity.

10. **You Have Arrived:** Ultimately, you need to have a positive mindset about exercise, especially aerobic exercise. When it becomes the high priority that it deserves to be, you have arrived! When you get to a level of fitness where you can easily distinguish between easy and hard exercise, you have arrived. There is nothing more enjoyable than to go for an easy (remember—this is a relative term) run, ride, swim, ski or row where you are able to shoot the breeze with your pals as you go, or just chill by yourself and take in your outdoor environment.

My favorite exercise at present is to go for an easy run on the Isle of Palms beach, sometimes alone, sometimes with friends, and just enjoy the sun, the sea, the sand, the wildlife—heaven! I remember the first time we went for a walk on the beach on Christmas Day. It was about 70 degrees, a beautiful sunny day, and we were very pleased with our decision to come to America. We rang our family back in Ireland as we walked and we could really sense the envy in their voices as we realized how lucky we were!

S—Strength

I am often asked which type of exercise is the most important of all. Sometimes it is presented with a time limitation like this—if I only have twenty minutes to exercise, what is the best way to spend my limited time? This is one situation where I truly believe that sitting on the fence is the best answer, because the right answer is that you really need to do each type of exercise as part of your overall exercise program.

We have already discussed **baseline** exercise and the importance of making it a much greater priority in your life. We also discussed **aerobic** exercise and I gave you ten reasons why I believe it is very important and must be included as an integral part of your weekly exercise program. We will discuss intensity, cross-training and stretching later but right now **strength** is in the spotlight and I intend to give it the level of priority it deserves.

You absolutely have to do muscle strengthening exercises and they should be a primary form of exercise along with your dominant form of exercise, which for most of you will be your aerobic activity of walking, running, swimming, biking, skiing, rowing, or whatever you choose to do.

Strength Exercises

Strength exercises can be done in a variety of ways. Some of you will think of weight training with machines in a gym or fitness center. You can also use free weights such as dumbbells or simply do exercises using your own body weight.

While I have done all forms of strength training over the years, my favorite form is to do simple strength exercise using my body weight and this is often referred to as circuit training. There are many reasons why. I can do these exercises anywhere and I nearly always do them outdoors. I don't need any special equipment and most importantly they are very functional; the exercises I do support my daily life, which at my age is what I need more than anything else!

Your goal should be to include two strength exercise sessions in your weekly exercise schedule. Starting off, this may be two fifteen-minute sessions a week, progressing slowly and gradually to two thirty-minute sessions. Eventually, you may get to two forty-five-minute sessions but most of us will not need to go beyond that.

Do Not Neglect Your Strength!

It is very easy to neglect your strength exercises and I know many people do. When runners get injured, more often than not, it is caused by the repetitive use of the same muscles with the corresponding relative neglect of their other muscles. Strengthening the muscles which stabilize your hips and knees in particular, is very important for injury prevention. Making weak muscles stronger will reduce imbalances which exist between opposing muscle groups. Instead of adding a fourth or fifth walk or run to your weekly training schedule, you will nearly always be better off in the long run, excuse the pun, to do some functional strength exercises instead. This is probably counterintuitive, which explains why so few runners practice it. However, perhaps the most interesting thing is that by adding strength exercises to your routine, your running will also improve.

Avoid Sarcopenia

One of the main reasons you have to do these functional strength exercises is because of the loss of muscle mass as you age, known as *sarcopenia*. This starts at about age thirty and continues at a rate of between 0.5% to 1% a year. This rate accelerates in your late fifties and early sixties, unless you take action to avoid it.

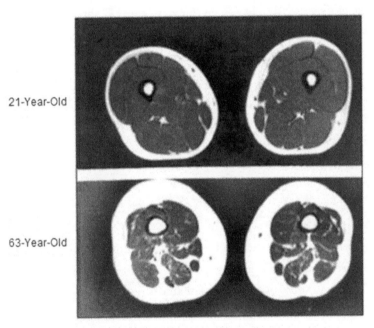

Age-related changes in muscle mass in thigh cross-sectional area of two people with similar BMI.

The picture above shows the huge difference between the muscle mass of the thigh of an average twenty-one year-old compared to a sixty-three year-old. This change in muscle mass is what typically happens to the average American, but it doesn't have to be like this! If you exercise regularly and include two muscle strengthening sessions a week in your exercise program, you can significantly postpone this process.

Your Metabolism

Strength exercises will also boost your metabolism, which means you will burn energy more efficiently, which in turn will help you control or lose weight. In addition, as you increase your muscle mass and slow down sarcopenia you actually burn more calories; each additional pound of muscle burns calories approximately three times faster than fat. It may not be hugely significant, but it all helps in the fight against illness and aging.

I—Intensity

High intensity exercise should be an integral part of your weekly training program. While cardio or aerobic exercise is great, it is not effective in the longer-term if that is all you do. Just like strength exercises in the last section, you should exercise at different levels of intensity. That is how you at least maintain your current strength and fitness levels. Preferably, however, you will get even fitter, stronger and faster. By doing so, your health benefits will increase and your life expectancy and quality of life will improve. Also, like strength exercises, high intensity exercise will boost your metabolism; you will burn energy more efficiently, which will help you lose or control your weight.

Take Care When Starting

As you might imagine, you need to be careful with high intensity workouts. If you try to do too much too quickly, you are just asking for trouble. You will greatly increase your risk of injury and that will defeat the whole purpose of doing higher intensity workouts in the first place.

If you are just starting out or trying to get back into exercise after a long period of inactivity, you really do not need to worry about high intensity exercise. Your first priority is to gradually build your fitness level by doing aerobic exercise, not high intensity stuff. The aerobic activity you do at the start will provide all the challenge you need in the early months of this process. There will be plenty of time to introduce higher intensity exercise later.

Importance of Rest and Recovery

Three or four months back into regular exercise, your fitness level will be significantly enhanced. While your workouts will still be relatively hard, it is not a good idea to work hard every day. Your body needs time to recover. There are two ways to do this—one is to rest completely and the other is to have an "easy" day or recovery day, which means your workload is relatively easy, compared to a hard day.

Some fitness "experts" recommend that your focus should be on high intensity exercise only and that you need do no more than, say, fifteen to twenty minutes, three times a week—a total of about one hour of exercise a week. They argue that a major bonus to their approach is the significant time saved by not having to do "very time-consuming and boring" aerobic exercise, which they increasingly present as both a "chore and a waste of time". While this approach may become increasingly popular with those who like to take short cuts, as previously stated, in my view, it is wrong and there is much evidence to support my view.

Copy the Professionals

There isn't a professional or elite athlete on the planet who doesn't have a complete training program which includes the following:

- Warm-up, which is cardio or aerobic exercise
- Flexibility or stretching exercises
- Stride outs, which are faster aerobic exercises in preparation for higher intensity
- Speed workout at high intensity, usually with slower aerobic activity between intervals
- Cool down, which is cardio or aerobic exercise with more stretching exercises

Now, you don't have to do exactly what professional or elite athletes do but it surely makes sense to mimic the principles that they employ. This will take more time than high intensity exercise alone, but there is simply no way around it. Since this is the case, it is all the more important that you should enjoy that time, have fun and minimize your risk of injury. As you can see, I have nothing against high intensity exercise but I believe it should be part of your overall exercise plan.

While harder, more intensive exercise sessions are just that—harder and more intensive—they provide a great sense of achievement, especially when you can see that you are making progress. There are many different types of high intensity exercise that you can do.

Interval Training

This is often referred to as speed-work by athletes. It is usually done at a running track, though it doesn't have to be. Let me give you an example: after warming up for at least ten minutes, you run or fast walk (4 x 400m), which is four times around the track with a two to three minute rest between your intervals. A slightly more difficult twist on this is to slowly jog rather than rest between repeats.

You should always cool down with an easy ten minute walk or run before you finish. This is a great way to introduce higher intensity exercise into your workouts, so that you can start slowly and gradually build up intensity. Of course, you can do intervals for swimming, biking, skiing, kayaking, etc. as well.

Fartlek

This is a Swedish term for speed-play. It blends high intensity intervals and aerobic exercise. So, for example, you go for a thirty minute walk, run, swim or ride starting at a comfortable pace. After warming up for ten minutes, you speed up for one minute, then slow down for one minute, speed up for one minute and you continue the process for ten minutes before you cool down for the final ten minutes. This is another great way to introduce higher intensity workouts into your exercise and is very easy to do.

Tempo

This is where you increase the intensity of your exercise for a longer period, often to mimic racing conditions. So, for example, a runner training for a 5K road race might include a two or three mile tempo run in preparation for the race. As always, you should warm up before tempo runs and cool down after them.

Hills

Any exercise which involves going up hills automatically increases intensity, so they are another great way to increase the intensity of your training. Of course, you need to pick your hills carefully, so you do not bite off more than you can chew. The same principles of warming up and cooling down apply.

Intensity As You Get Older

As you get older, you can make considerable progress doing higher intensity workouts, though it should be seen for what it is. While long-term your body may be slowing down, in the short-term you will be getting faster and thus making progress. This is a key concept to wrap your head around, because you will eventually slow down as you age, but hopefully you will do so gradually and over a long period of time.

Unless you are a very serious and advanced athlete, in my view, you should do no more than two high intensity training sessions a week. In fact, as you get older, one may be enough, unless you are in serious training for a race. You always have to listen to your body and make sure you, and not your ego, are in control.

As I am not racing at present, I don't do as much higher intensity training as I used to, but I still try to get in one session a week. I usually do 400 or 800 meter repeats on my local track, or if I decide to go longer I will run on the ashfelt path beside the track, which is a little easier on my joints.

C—Cross Training

While I love running, in the longer term it is not a good idea to only run. As previously mentioned, this is because eventually the repetitive usage of the same muscles can lead to injury, usually caused by the relative weaknesses in the muscles you do not use as often. This is true of most dominant activities you do such as walking, running, cycling, rowing or whatever. However, it is fair to say that some exercises are better than others. For example, swimming uses many different muscles, but there is little wear and tear on your joints.

As discussed earlier, you absolutely must do muscle strengthening exercises and they really should be a fundamental part of your weekly exercise right along with your dominant exercise. For example, running is my dominant form of exercise at present and I also do two strength exercise sessions each week. We also discussed the importance of introducing higher intensity exercise into your weekly exercise.

Introduce Another Form of Exercise

As you increase the amount of time you spend exercising each week, it is also a very good idea to cross-train. Cross-training is simply a technical term which means that you should do other forms of exercise along with your dominant exercise. So instead of, say, running four or five days a week, you introduce a different form of exercise in place of one or two of your runs. In doing this, the cross-training should usually replace your low priority, easy run days. Exercises such as swimming and biking are great cross-training activities.

This new cross-training activity will provide welcome variety in your workouts and increase the overall enjoyment of your exercise, which should be an important, ongoing objective. If you are competitive, cross-training allows you to train a bit harder because while you may be using the same muscles, they are being used differently. Also, cross-training gives you a break, or what you might call an "active rest day" and this helps you recover faster from your higher intensity days.

So, cross-training is a great way to really promote optimum fitness. Other great forms of cross-training you should try if you get a chance are skiing, kayaking or rowing, yoga, Pilates and triathlon.

The Growth of Triathlon

Anyone can run and ride a bike, and a majority of people can swim, so when you start cross-training with one of these activities, you are actively doing two of the three components of a triathlon. It is therefore not really a huge leap to add the third ingredient; this is one of the reasons why triathlon has become so popular over the last twenty years.

I know, some of you are thinking, "this guy is crazy" but truly, you should not be put off by my reference to triathlon. Most triathletes are either runners, cyclists or swimmers who decided to cross-train and then said, "Hey, I may as well go whole hog and do a triathlon!" The vast majority of triathletes do what is called a sprint triathlon, which is a 750m swim followed by a 20k bike ride and a 5k run. It is without doubt a great feat to do any triathlon but for most people, it takes less time to complete a sprint triathlon than a half marathon.

Only a small number of participants who complete a sprint triathlon ever progress to the next level of triathlon, which is an Olympic-distance triathlon.

The official distance is exactly twice that of the sprint-distance triathlon. This is what is raced at the Olympic Games—hence the name Olympic-distance triathlon. An even smaller number of participants progress to complete the Ironman or half Ironman triathlons. These are much longer endurance events and for many, myself included, the investment of time required is too great!

I was a runner for nearly twenty years before I did my first triathlon. I was a reasonable swimmer from all those summers at Blackrock Baths (see Chapter 3), but the last time I had ridden a bike with any regularity was also back in those summers, when I was in my early teens.

Then, some twenty-five years later, during the early nineties, a group of my Irish friends, affectionately known as "the lads", decided to go on a cycling trip to Cork and Kerry in the southwest of Ireland. We had such a fantastic time that it became an annual trip and the cycling was great, too! On one of those trips, one night over a few pints of Guinness, a few of us agreed to do a triathlon. I was the only one who followed through and the next summer I did my first triathlon.

S—Stretching

It is not unusual to see runners stretching before they exercise. I am sure you can all picture them stretching their calf muscles against a tree or their hamstring with one foot on the trunk of their car. Is stretching good for you? Should you stretch before you exercise? Should you stretch after you exercise? Should you do both? What is correct stretching? What is incorrect stretching? Many questions—let's answer them.

Stretching Is Not Warming Up

Some people stretch before exercise and have done so for many years. I am not a fan of stretching before exercise unless you are properly warmed up in advance. Done properly, gentle, focused stretching or active dynamic stretching is good *after* warming up for at least ten minutes of easy walking or running. But beware—stretching a cold muscle can damage it if the stretch is too much!

Stretching after exercise is definitely a good idea. By doing this you improve the flexibility of muscles that would otherwise have stiffened and tightened up after exercise and this will pay immediate dividends in your next workout. It is especially beneficial for runners, for flexibility of the ankles, calves, hamstrings and hips is important in improving performance and avoiding injury.

What is Proper Stretching?

Stretching is definitely good for you when done correctly. I prefer the term flexibility because everyone can see the sense of maintaining good flexibility and it doesn't carry any negative baggage, though essentially it amounts to the same thing.

The greater your flexibility, the better your range of motion, and this will positively influence your performance. Unfortunately, when stretching is done incorrectly, it can do more harm than good. As not many people know how to stretch properly, there is a real risk of injury involved here.

Like most things, there is a right way and a wrong way to stretch. The wrong way, which is unfortunately practiced by many, is to bounce up and down, or to stretch to the point of pain. These methods can be harmful and often result in injury. Another approach I often see, which is simply a waste of time, is very short stretches which last no more than ten or fifteen seconds.

The right way is a relaxed, sustained stretch of at least thirty seconds, during which time your attention is focused on the muscle being stretched. You should never experience pain; if you do you should stop right away and get the ice out!

Why Stretch?

Regular stretching will provide the following benefits:

- It reduces muscle tension and relaxes your body
- It improves your coordination through freer and easier movement
- It increases your range of motion
- It helps to prevent injuries
- It is a quiet period of time out, which is good for thinking

Think about stretching this way. If you have ever been injured, what is the first thing you are told to do when rehabilitating your injury? The answer is to improve your flexibility and increase your muscle strength.

Stretching feels good when it is done properly. You should definitely not see it as a competitive part of your training; it should not be a personal contest to see how far you can stretch. The keys to stretching are regularity and relaxation. Your aim should be to reduce muscular tension and promote freer movement—not to focus on extreme stretching which can lead to injuries.

So, why do most of us only stretch when we are injured? I think the answer is time. This applies to stretching in the same way that it applies to strength exercises. We tend to say to ourselves, "I don't have time to do everything, and since I don't have any problems right now, I don't really need to stretch." Thus, we cut out the things that we believe are less important. This line of thinking works in the short-term, but unfortunately it will probably, over the longer-term, come back to haunt you.

✗ Your "To Do" List

1. If you are just starting out or returning to exercise after a layoff, your initial focus should be on these four elements of the B.A.S.I.C.S: **Baseline + Aerobic + Strength + Stretching.**

2. As you progress through the 5 Progressive Levels of Exercise, you should gradually introduce higher intensity exercise and cross-training.

3. Take immediate daily action to increase your Baseline exercise; this is especially important if you spend a lot of your typical day sitting.

4. For your exercise to truly be your secret sauce, it should include each element of the B.A.S.I.C.S.

"There are no shortcuts to any place worth going."
—Beverly Sills

CHAPTER 10

HOW TO ALLOCATE YOUR EXERCISE TIME

n Chapter 8, I answered the question about how *long* should you spend exercising. I also explained the important distinction between how *long* you spend exercising and how to measure how *much* exercise you should do. And, as you will remember, how much exercise is a better measure, because it takes both the quantity (time) and quality (intensity) of your exercise into account.

In Chapter 9, I answered the question of what *type* of exercise you should do and I introduced you to the B.A.S.I.C.S. We now need to pull all this information together and answer the ultimate question:

How should you allocate your exercise time between each kind of exercise?
The table below answers this question by providing a summary allocation of your exercise time. Remember—this table should be used as a general guideline and is not meant to be seen as precise. Also, remember that your planned exercise time

does not include baseline exercise and you should do as much baseline exercise as you can every day.

Summary Allocation of Your Exercise Time

	Level 1	Level 2	Level 3	Level 4	Level 5
Days/Week	4	5	5	5	6
Hours/Week	3	4	5	6	7
Primary Aerobic Activity	Walk	Walk/ Run	V Slow Run	Slow Run	Run
Aerobic Time	150	210	225	230	240
Strength Time	30	30	45	60	60
High Intensity Time	0	0	30	40	60
Cross-training Time	0	0	0	30	60
Total Time— Minutes	180	240	300	360	420
Avg. Intensity (METS)	3.3	5.0	6.0	6.7	7.1
Total Energy— MET Mins.	600	1200	1800	2400	3000

Note: Some people call slow or very slow running "jogging". However to me, the definition of jogging is an easy run, and as slow running is usually not very easy when starting out, I prefer to call it what it is—slow running.

The above table shows my weekly recommendations for days and hours of exercise at each level. It also shows my preferred primary aerobic activities, which begin with walking at Level 1 and progress to running in Level 2 and beyond. This is because both are relatively easy to do and because running is my favorite exercise, after all! However, if you prefer swimming, biking, cross-country skiing or whatever, that is absolutely fine with me. The key here is that you build a healthy exercise program into your life!

Your total exercise time is allocated to each kind of exercise, with aerobic activity getting the most for two reasons: First, because cardio is so important to your overall health and second, because you can only allocate so much time to strength and high intensity training. You will notice that I have not allocated any time to stretching, but it is still very important to include this in your daily exercise routine.

Time to Reach Level 5

You do not have to get to the top of Level 5 in any specific timeframe. There are no rules about how long you should take; essentially you should take as long as you need to, taking your specific set of circumstances into account. Nonetheless, I have created the graph below to act as a general guide.

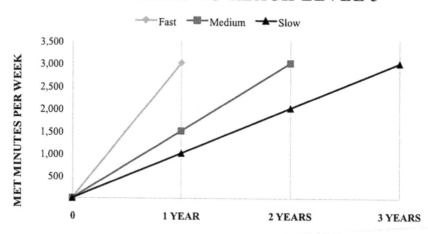

The fast track to Level 5 is one year and the slow track is three years, with everything else in between. It's up to you to decide the appropriate track for you based on your own personal circumstances. If you are already active, you need to find the starting level that is right for you.

The increase in weekly energy expenditure from Level 1 (600 METS) to Level 5 (3000 METS) is significant—Level 5 uses five times more energy than Level 1. While progression through each level is designed to be challenging, it is also very realistic and well within the scope of most adults. You should only start a new level when you are comfortably able to complete the level on which you currently are.

5X Fitness Transformation

I have developed a comprehensive fitness program called 5X Fitness Transformation, or 5XFT for short. 5XFT is based on my Exercise BASICS Formula and designed so you can ease into the best shape of your life, regardless of your age, weight or current fitness level.

It is called 5XFT for two important reasons. The five represents the 5 Progressive Levels of Exercise and the X represents the progression that you will experience on your journey. As you progress from Level 1 to Level 2 you use 2X the weekly energy expenditure, all the way up to 5X at Level 5.

Level 1 is the right starting point if you have been inactive for some time (three months or more) and you want to ease yourself back into exercise. Level 2 is the right starting point if you are already exercising at least three hours a week. To put this another way, you would be well able to complete Level 1 and thus Level 2 is an appropriate progression for you. The same principles apply through Levels 3, 4 and 5.

If you follow 5XFT, your new lifestyle journey will truly be a "Transformation" from where you are today. 5XFT is *not* a quick fix; it is about transforming your lifestyle. Moreover—and this is a **crucial point**—it will take you *at least* a year to complete all 5 Levels:

52 Weeks To Level 5

Here is an approximation of how long it should take you to master each level:

- Level 1 - 9 Weeks
- Level 2 - 9 Weeks
- Level 3 - 12 Weeks
- Level 4 - 12 Weeks
- Level 5 - 10 Weeks

5XFT is an investment in your new lifestyle, your life expectancy and the future quality of your life. You will make remarkable progress on your journey and ultimately *you will transform your life.* There is no going back to your old lifestyle, with little or no exercise. Your new journey has only started and exercise, with all its benefits, will be your "secret sauce", a high priority for the rest of your life. If you would like to find out more about 5XFT go to **www.GetAmericaMoving. com/5XFT**.

✗ Your "To Do" List

1. Using the table at the start of this chapter to guide you, develop a plan to allocate your time between each kind of exercise.

2. Taking your current fitness and your personal circumstances into account, decide at what level you need to start and how long it will take you to get to Level 5.

3. Review the summary page for each level in the remaining pages of this chapter and consider whether 5XFT can help, support, motivate and inspire you on your journey.

> *"You have only one life, and no one else will*
> *live it for you. Shouldn't you take the time right now*
> *to figure out what that life is all about?"*
> **—Harry Browne**

5XFT Level 1 Summary

If you are currently inactive, you should start at 5XFT Level 1 and gradually work your way through the nine week fitness program. You will find step-by-step, day-by-day, week-by-week instructions, with all the supporting information you need, in the 5XFT Level 1 eBook and videos.

It is important as you work your way through Level 1 that you can get back into the habit of exercise, having some fun and building your confidence along the way. 5XFT Level 1 gradually builds up to 600 MET Minutes of energy expenditure per week, which is consistent with Level 1 of the *Physical Activity Guidelines for Americans*.

When you complete Level 1, you will be able to do 3 hours of moderate intensity exercise a week, made up of 150 minutes of moderate walking and 30 minutes of muscle strengthening. The average intensity is 3.33 METS, for a total of 600 MET Minutes per week as set out in the table below.

Weekly Exercise Summary	5XFT Level 1
Primary Aerobic Activity	**Moderate Walking**
1. Exercise Time (in Minutes)	150
Average Intensity (METS)	3.33
MET Minutes	500
2. Muscle Strengthening Time	30
Average Intensity (METS)	3.33
MET Minutes	100
3. Total Time (in Minutes)	180
Overall Average Intensity	3.33
Total MET Minutes	600

5XFT Level 2 Summary

Before you progress to 5XFT Level 2, you should be able to exercise comfortably at the top of Level 1 for 4 weeks. It is important to understand that you do not progress to the top of Level 2 in one go. Like all things relating to exercise, your progress should be gradual and spaced evenly over the nine week fitness program. You will find step-by-step, day-by-day, week-by-week instructions for Level 2, along with all the supporting information you need, in the 5XFT Level 2 eBook and videos.

By the time you complete Level 2, your weekly energy expenditure will have increased to 1200 MET Minutes. That is twice the energy expenditure of Level 1, which is a significant increase. In order to achieve this, you will need to increase both your weekly exercise time and intensity. Your overall time increases by one hour to four hours per week and your muscle strengthening gradually increases to a more vigorous intensity of 6.67 METS. The average intensity of your other exercise increases gradually from 3.33 to 4.76 METS. Over a nine week period, this is very realistic.

Weekly Exercise Summary	5XFT Level 1	5XFT Level 2
Primary Aerobic Activity	**Moderate Walking**	**Walk/Run**
1. Exercise Time (Minutes)	150	210
Average Intensity (METS)	3.33	4.76
MET Minutes	500	1000
2. Muscle Strengthening Time	30	30
Average Intensity	3.33	6.67
MET Minutes	100	200
3. Total Time (Minutes)	180	240
Overall Average Intensity	3.33	5.0
Total MET Minutes	600	1200

5XFT Level 3 Summary

Before you progress to 5XFT Level 3, you should be able to comfortably complete Level 2. It is important to understand that you do not progress to the top of Level 3 in one go. Like all things relating to exercise, your progress should be gradual and spaced over the twelve week fitness program. You will find step-by-step, day-by-day, week-by-week instructions for Level 3, with all the supporting information you need, in the 5XFT Level 3 eBook and videos.

By the time you complete Level 3, your weekly energy expenditure will have increased to 1800 MET Minutes. That is an additional 600 MET Minutes – the equivalent of Levels 1 and 2 combined. This is a significant increase and to achieve this, you will need to increase both your weekly exercise time and intensity. Your overall time increases by one hour to five hours per week, which includes forty-five minutes of muscle strengthening done at an average intensity of 6.67 METS. The average intensity of your other exercise increases from 4.8 to 5.9 METS and over a twelve week period, this is very realistic. Remember—if you start at Level 1, it will take you at least eighteen weeks to get to the start of 5XFT Level 3.

Weekly Exercise Summary	5XFT Level 2	5XFT Level 3
Primary Aerobic Activity	**Walk/Run**	**Very Slow Run**
1. Exercise Time (Minutes)	210	255
Average Intensity (METS)	4.76	5.9
MET Minutes	1000	1500
2. Muscle Strengthening Time	30	45
Average Intensity	6.7	6.7
MET Minutes	200	300
3. Total Time (Minutes)	240	300
Overall Average Intensity	5.0	6.0
Total MET Minutes	1200	1800

5XFT Level 4 Summary

Before you progress to 5XFT Level 4, you should be able to comfortably complete Level 3. It is important to understand that you do not progress to the top of Level 4 in one go. Like all things relating to exercise, your progress should be gradual and spaced over the twelve week fitness program. You will find step-by-step, day-by-day, week-by-week instructions for 5XFT Level 4, along with all the supporting information you need, in the 5XFT Level 4 eBook and videos.

By the time you complete 5XFT Level 4, your weekly energy expenditure will have increased to 2400 MET Minutes. That is an additional 600 MET Minutes, which is a significant increase. In order to achieve this, you will need to increase both your weekly exercise time and intensity. Your overall time increases by one hour to six hours per week; this includes one hour of muscle strengthening, which remains at an average intensity of 6.67 METS. The average intensity of your other exercise increases from 5.8 to 6.7 METS and over a twelve week period, this is very realistic. Remember—if you start at Level 1, it will take you at least thirty weeks to get to the start of 5XFT Level 4.

Weekly Exercise Summary	5XFT Level 3	5XFT Level 4
Primary Aerobic Activity	Very Slow Run	Slow Run
1. Exercise Time (Minutes)	260	300
Average Intensity (METS)	5.77	6.7
MET Minutes	1500	2000
2. Muscle Strengthening Time	40	60
Average Intensity	7.5	6.7
MET Minutes	300	400
3. Total Time	300	360
Overall Average Intensity	6.0	6.7
Total MET Minutes	1800	2400

5XFT Level 5 Summary

Before you progress to 5XFT Level 5, you should be able to comfortably complete Level 4. It is important to understand that you do not progress to the top of Level 5 in one go. Like all things relating to exercise, your progress should be gradual and spaced over the ten week fitness program. You will find step-by-step, day-by-day, week-by-week instructions for Level 5, along with all the supporting information you need, in the 5XFT Level 5 eBook and videos.

By the time you complete 5XFT Level 5, your weekly energy expenditure will have increased to 3000 MET Minutes. That is an additional 600 MET Minutes, which is a significant increase. In order to achieve this, you will need to increase both your weekly exercise time and intensity. Your overall time increases by one hour to seven hours per week; this includes one hour of muscle strengthening, which increases to a more vigorous average intensity of 7.5 METS. The average intensity of your other exercise increases from 6.7 to 7.1 METS and over a ten week period, this is very realistic. Remember—if you start at Level 1, it will take you at least forty-two weeks to get to the start of 5XFT Level 5.

Weekly Exercise Summary	5XFT Level 4	5XFT Level 5
Primary Aerobic Activity	**Slow Run**	**Run**
1. Exercise Time (Minutes)	300	360
Average Intensity (METS)	6.7	7.1
MET Minutes	2000	2550
2. Muscle Strengthening Time	60	60
Average Intensity	6.7	7.5
MET Minutes	400	450
3. Total Time	360	420
Overall Average Intensity	6.7	7.1
Total MET Minutes	2400	3000

PART 3

TURBOCHARGE YOUR LIFE
WITH THE X FACTOR

INTRODUCTION TO PART 3

In Part 3 of *The eXercise Factor* I reveal the X Factor and the five essential stages that you will need to follow if you want to increase your life expectancy and improve your quality of life.

In **Chapter 11**, I will introduce you to the X Man exercise and the acronym R.E.C.I.P.E.—the six key ingredients of the X Factor. Finally, before we move on to the next chapter, I will reveal what the X Factor stands for.

In **Chapter 12**, we discuss the first essential stage that you need to follow. I have called this chapter Your X Factor Decision because I don't want to reveal what it represents here in the introduction.

In **Chapter 13,** Your Current Fitness Level, we discuss your second essential stage for success. You need a clear understanding of your current fitness level because this is your starting position. You will record some key health measures, your current exercise details and you will complete your one mile fitness challenge so you can select your appropriate starting level.

In **Chapter 14**, we discuss your third essential step, Your Project Plan. You will develop a plan for your first project using another important acronym P.R.O.J.E.C.T.—to guide you.

In **Chapter 15**, we discuss your fourth essential step—Your Project Implementation. We will discuss the importance of project execution and of recording key project information.

In **Chapter 16**, we discuss your fifth and final essential step—Your Project Review. This includes the importance of celebrating and rewarding your success and then taking your time before you select your next project.

CHAPTER 11

THE X FACTOR REVEALED

n Chapter 5, I introduced you to the 4 Key Drivers of Success. These are the key ingredients which you need to genuinely focus on if you want to succeed and have a long, happy, healthy life. As a quick reminder, the first driver is knowledge, about each of the other ingredients and especially about your health. Part 4 is devoted to knowledge. The second ingredient is nutrition and you need to educate yourself and implement healthy eating and drinking initiatives on an ongoing basis. Chapter 19 in Part 4 is about nutrition. The third key driver or ingredient is exercise, the secret sauce to a long, high quality life. Part 2 was devoted to the importance of exercise.

The fourth key driver works very closely alongside the other three drivers, especially exercise, and really pulls everything together. I call this driver the X Factor and in many respects it is the most important ingredient of all. That is why I called the book *The eXercise Factor*. If you have this key ingredient you are very likely to succeed but without it, you are doomed to failure. While there are no guarantees, with the X Factor you are very likely to enjoy a significant increase in both your life expectancy and the quality of your life.

The X Man Exercise

How do you know if you have the X Factor and how do you ensure you have it in the future? To help answer these questions, I would like to introduce you to the X Man logo that started my new life in America back in 2003. Affectionately known as "the X Man" to TrySports staff back then, I still use the X Man as a metaphor to help folks understand the importance of the X Factor to a long and healthy lifestyle.

There is a direct relationship between the X Man logo and the X Factor and I have referenced it often when speaking to groups such as the Healthy Charleston Challenge. As previously mentioned, the Challenge is Charleston's version of *The Biggest Loser* television competition—in fact, by joining the Challenge the participants have already made an important decision to change their lives. I usually speak to them when they only have a few weeks to go and when they need to start thinking of life beyond the Challenge. So I show them the X Man and I ask them what they see and what the X Man is saying to them. This usually gets a very positive and fruitful response from the Challenge participants. Before I reveal the typical answers on the next page, why not take a few minutes, have a good look at the X Man below and ask yourself the same questions. Write your thoughts down before you look at the answers on the next page.

Welcome back! How did you get on? When asking an audience about what the X Man logo means to them, I always get plenty of suggestions, some good and some not so good, but the most common, relevant ideas are as follows:

- **Crossroads:** You are at a crossroads and you have a choice of directions or paths; you have to decide which direction you wish to take.
- **Journey**: Like contestants on *The Biggest Loser* or participants in the Healthy Charleston Challenge, you are on a voyage of discovery, a journey which for many of you may only be starting.
- **Sun, Moon or Star:** To look down on you and guide you on your voyage or to act as a goal or target for your future journey.

I hope these ideas makes sense to you. Now that you are thinking this way, it should be easy for you to make the link between your past, your present and your future. I always try to get the Healthy Charleston Challenge participants to really start thinking about their future journey once the Challenge is over.

The Challenge has been an amazing voyage for the participants and in the vast majority of cases it is categorically a positive experience and catalyst for their new lifestyle. They have started their journey and I heavily emphasize the fact that they have already made their decision and that there is no going back. While they have just experienced a life-changing event, their true voyage of discovery has only just begun.

They still have some important decisions ahead as they continue the journey that has already started to change their lives. By continuing to make the right choices and take the right actions regarding their health, nutrition and exercise, they will enrich their new lifestyle, increase their life expectancy and improve their quality of life by significantly reducing illness and injury, and significantly delaying symptoms associated with so-called "normal" aging.

Your Future Journey

Like the Healthy Charleston Challenge participants, you too should be ready to make the jump from the X Man logo metaphor to thinking about your future. You also have a decision to make, a path to take, a new journey to travel. This is not just about your health, nutrition and exercise—it is about a new challenge and a new lifestyle. You need to be highly motivated to succeed, so how do you do this? How can you maximize your chances of success?

The X Factor Exercise

To help you think about and understand what I mean by the X Factor, I have created the simple acronym R.E.C.I.P.E. which describes six key ingredients. If these ingredients are present, your chances of success will soar. Can you guess what each letter stands for?

Just like a cake, when these ingredients are combined they make up the X Factor. Take some time out now and see if you can figure out what each of the six letters stands for.

Nobody has ever gotten all six correct. If you can get three or more right you are doing very well. However, what is much more important than this task is that you feel—no, you believe—that you either possess some of these elements already or that you are determined to develop them. If you do, then you are well on your way to possessing the X Factor. So take ten or fifteen minutes, using the space provided below to record your thoughts before turning the page.

R =

E =

C =

I =

P =

E =

Welcome back! How did you get on? I hope you found the exercise helpful. Now look below to see how many you got right. If you didn't get the precise words, I am sure you were thinking along similar lines.

RECIPE—Six Key Ingredients of the X Factor

When presenting live, I always reveal the 6 ingredients one by one, describing each one as I go and giving out prizes to those who get the right answers. This creates a build-up of anticipation and keeps everyone actively involved before I reveal what the X Factor stands for. There—I have just given you one of the 6 ingredients!

Unfortunately, I cannot follow that approach here so I will start by first giving you all 6 ingredients together so that you can check them against your answers. Then I will go through them one by one before I finally reveal what the X Factor stands for. I am sure the suspense is killing you at this stage but be patient—it won't be long now!

R—**Resolve**

E—**Energetic**

C—**Cause**

I—**Involved**

P—**Projects**

E—**Extraordinary**

R—Resolve

Have you the resolve necessary to change your lifestyle? Are you resilient enough to persevere through the hard times, especially at the beginning? Are you committed enough to make this happen?

These are some pretty tough questions that force you to search your soul about your true future intentions. Do you *really* want to change? In order for this to work, you will need to be fully committed to your new challenge and lifestyle. You have some very important questions to answer and decisions to make if you want to succeed. Before you move on you need to make two key decisions as follows:

1. Where does exercise fit into your priorities?
2. Are you prepared to allocate the time required to adapt to your new lifestyle?

In their book *Performance-Driven Thinking,* authors David Hancock and Bobby Kipper define performance-driven thinking as "the thought process that connects the desire to perform with the will to perform a specific task or goal."[8] *Desire* is to long or hope for something you want, whereas *will* is to decide, attempt or bring desire to action. This is a very important distinction and it applies to the X Factor.

Your answers to the above questions will tell you whether you have the resolve to take the actions you need to take—whether you have the will to succeed in your new lifestyle.

E—Energetic

Whatever you decide to do, you will need to bring lots of positive energy and enthusiasm to the table on a sustained basis if you want to succeed. It is usually relatively easy to find a burst of energy at the start but as time moves on and the novelty wears off, it becomes increasingly difficult to maintain your momentum. That is why it is especially important that you choose something that you will enjoy.

In an ideal world, you should choose something that you have enjoyed in the past. Even better would be if you could rekindle something that you were, at one time, passionate about. If that option doesn't exist then try to choose something that you feel you can grow into and hopefully become both energetic and passionate about over time.

It is definitely possible for you to develop a passion for something new, and when you do, much positive energy will flow with it. A good example of this is running. Now I acknowledge that I am a little biased—no, let's just say that as a regular runner, I *am* biased. Some of you are probably thinking, "Is he crazy?" Others may be saying, "Over my dead body!" But please, give me a little latitude to explain.

---

8   David Hancock and Bobby Kipper, *Performance-Driven Thinking* (New York: Morgan James Publishing, 2014) pg. 7

For many people who are new to running, initially it can seem very hard and few really enjoy it at the start. You may even have to work hard to convince yourself that you like running at all. Some will describe it as no fun, even boring—especially when they do it by themselves. This makes it hard to be passionate about it, never mind energetic or enthusiastic.

However, about a year after starting, as I mentioned in Chapter 3 under the heading "Control", the vast majority of runners who had the resolve and energy to stick with it will, when they look back at their journey, describe it as one they really enjoyed. You would also be amazed at how many of them will say that they are now passionate about their running.

This is an important point, not just about running but about all exercise. Even now, despite my energy and my passion for exercise and running in particular, I still have some bad days and I just want to finish as quickly as I can. Most runners will tell you that going through the process described above is partly why they are now so energetic and enthusiastic about their new passion. In a sense, they earned the right to it and they are able to fondly look back and see how they developed it. You can do likewise, but you have to be energetic and have the courage to believe that you also can reach the Promised Land.

If you are a running skeptic, try to keep an open mind and make sure you read Chapter 21—Anyone Can Run.

C—Cause

Do you have a great cause which will inspire you to succeed? Finding a cause for your new lifestyle will significantly increase your chances of success. The more personal your cause, the better and having a great cause will keep you seriously motivated. If you can't think of a personal cause then thinking about your family, spouse, kids, grand-kids or partner usually does the trick.

Over the years, I have chosen many worthy causes to help me achieve my exercise goals. Coming from Ireland, our winters are long, wet, cold and generally miserable—not terribly conducive to exercising outdoors. As you know by now, I am very much a proponent of outdoor exercise, so finding a great cause was incredibly helpful.

To get me through the winters, I would always choose an event that I wanted to do the following spring. For example, in the fall of 1986, I decided I would do the London marathon the following May. I had just moved to live and work in London which, by the way, is much colder than Dublin in the winter. To help get me through the six or seven months of necessary training, I called the British Heart Foundation and asked them if they would like me to run for them. Of course, charities always say yes. And, as I worked in London's financial district at the time, I was able to raise a lot of money for my "cause".

I always got the paperwork (and it was actual paperwork back then) out of the way quickly. That way, barring injury, which only happened once, I was seriously motivated to achieve my goal and there was no way I was going to face the ignominy of failure. Nonetheless, to be completely honest, raising money for a cause that meant so much to me was an honor and I loved doing it. Look out for a similar story about the Clearwater triathlon later which has an interesting twist; it wasn't funny at the time, but it is now when I look back on it!

I—Involved

Are you prepared to really immerse yourself in your new lifestyle? The more involved you can get, the more likely you are to succeed. Having the necessary commitment to a task or goal is great, but involvement trumps commitment every time. Which reminds me of the bacon and eggs breakfast story; the hen is committed but the pig is involved!

So what do I mean by getting involved? The best way to illustrate this is with a few examples. In the illustration I gave you earlier, by choosing the British Heart Foundation I got involved in what was, for me, a major sponsorship campaign surrounding the completion of the marathon. By doing this, unless I got injured, I was never going to fail.

Another great example of involvement is the Healthy Charleston Challenge, which I mentioned at the start of this chapter. It is a powerful support mechanism and program for the participants. I often ask the participants if they think that they could have made the same progress without the Challenge. Inevitably, this helps them to understand the power of getting involved and taking action with the support, help, direction and supervision of coaches and mentors.

Likewise, participants in *The Biggest Loser* TV show will openly acknowledge that they could never have been as successful as they were without their coaches and all the support provided by the competition. It was their involvement in the competition which was the primary catalyst for their success.

Similarly, the members of a walking or running group who get involved will be the ones who are the most successful. Likewise, those who sign up for training programs to complete a race in the future invariably succeed and achieve their goals.

P—Projects

When you have a cause and you decide to get involved with a group of some kind, you essentially create a project. Projects will become foundational to the success of your new lifestyle, as illustrated in each of the examples provided above.

In my own case, by getting ***involved*** with the British Heart Foundation as my ***cause*** to help get me through my winter training for the London marathon, I essentially created a major ***project*** for 6 months of my life, which provided amazing memories that I will always cherish.

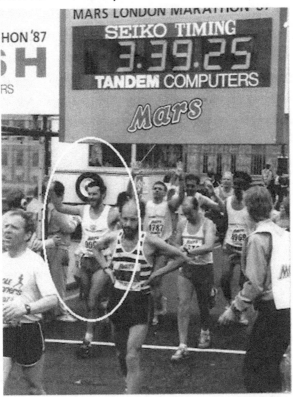

Let me introduce myself—the handsome guy with dark hair and beard to the left in the photo with my arms raised and a big smile on my face, despite the pain I was feeling. By the way, I could point out quite a few things that have changed: the cotton t-shirt, cotton socks, very short shorts, Tandem Computers—where have they gone?

They say photos cannot lie but let me tell you a story with which all runners will identify. The official time in this photo is the big lie, at least as far as I am concerned. It says I finished in 3:39:25, which is a respectable time for the marathon. However, I was actually about five minutes faster. There were some thirty-five thousand participants in the race that day and it took me just over five minutes to cross the starting line at the beginning of the race, so my real time was around 3:34:00.

It was an amazing start to the race, one which I will never forget. After finally crossing the starting line, it probably took me at least another ten minutes before I was running at my planned pace. I learned something very important that day about racing; by being forced to start very slowly, I was able to finish strong. Including the five minutes at the start, this was my best marathon time ever.

Likewise, the participants in the Healthy Charleston Challenge and *The Biggest Loser* competitions got involved with major projects of their own. And members of a walking or running group, by joining the group and signing up for training programs geared towards the completion of a road race, got themselves involved in projects.

Before we move on, there is one last point I would like to make about projects. As you move forward through your upcoming journey and your new lifestyle, you will go from strength to strength by getting involved in back-to-back projects. We will discuss projects in greater detail in Chapter 14.

E—Extraordinary

You could argue that the last ingredient of the X Factor is not really an ingredient at all. Rather, it is the result you will get when you roll the other five ingredients together. You need to have the **resolve** to change your life, especially at the start. If you can bring much **energy** to the table and combine this with activities about which you are either already passionate or feel you can become passionate, you are on the road to success.

If you can find a great *cause* which enables you to get fully ***involved*** in a major ***project*** which helps you achieve your objectives, you have all the ingredients to achieve ***extraordinary*** success and create the lifestyle you are seeking.

You can do this if you sincerely want to, but to succeed you must see all of this as a very high priority in your life, if not your highest. So at last we come to the answer to the question—what is the X Factor?

What is the X Factor?

The X Factor is your MISSION! It is your new challenge, your new journey, your voyage of discovery—in other words: **You need to be on a mission!**

My choice of the word "mission" has been probably forty years in the making and has been influenced by many different parts of my life including:

- Twenty-five years working in personnel management
- Twenty-four years as an entrepreneur
- Ten years as the owner and CEO of TrySports
- Forty years as a runner, triathlete and coach
- My new mission as creator of Get America Moving

I believe it is an appropriate choice of words because one way or another, whether you like it or not, you are on a mission. I also believe it makes sense to control your destiny and you can do this when you know what your mission is!

Like me, I'm sure you want to live a long and healthy life. When I was in my twenties, living into my seventies seemed like a great deal, especially since my dad died at forty-seven and my mum died at sixty-seven. However, now that I am close to sixty, this doesn't seem like such a great deal any more. As I get older, I keep adjusting my target, which I suppose is a pretty natural thing to do. I am now thinking into my nineties, and who knows? With my mission, maybe even a hundred is possible. That would give me at least another thirty to forty years; that's more like it!

No Guarantees

Of course, I could drop dead tomorrow. I know there are no guarantees and because of that I am seriously motivated to do everything I can to achieve my mission. While I cannot control the outcome, I can influence the process and there are a multitude of things I can do to increase my chances of not just achieving the quantitative target, but doing so in a qualitative way. What I mean by that is I want to make sure that those additional years are really worth living—that I am fit and healthy enough to thoroughly enjoy my remaining time here.

When I think this way about my fitness and health, while it is still not *easy*, it is much *easier* to find the high levels of motivation required to be successful on my mission. For me, this is a voyage which will last a long time—a lifetime! If you are thinking along similar lines, I invite you to join me on this extraordinary journey. At TrySports, we had a motto: "Get Fit, Stay Fit, Live Fit". This is not a marketing tagline; it is serious business!

You Have Two Options

Consequently, one way or another your current lifestyle determines how long and healthy your life will be. Essentially you have two options: you can choose to face your problems and take action to solve them or you can continue down the path you are currently on, which will inevitably lead to a deterioration of your health, with chronic illness and injury for many years.

Stay on the same path and you will significantly increase your risk of heart disease, diabetes, obesity, dementia including Alzheimer's, stress, sleep apnea and depression. The list goes on and on, so unless you take action, you will experience a much lower quality of life, much higher healthcare costs and ultimately a much earlier death.

The other option is to take action. You <u>can</u> overcome your personal health and fitness problems and develop a new sustainable, long-term way of living. Most important of all, you <u>can</u> succeed and get to where you would like to be and achieve your dreams.

Improve Your Health

Positive action will facilitate a dramatic improvement in your health, especially if:

- You would like to significantly reduce the risk of heart disease and improve key health markers such as your blood pressure, cholesterol, triglycerides and blood sugar.
- You are overweight or obese and you would like to achieve normal weight.
- You have diabetes or pre-diabetes and would like to get rid of it.
- You want to significantly reduce your risk of Alzheimer's disease and other forms of dementia as you get older.

Inspire Others

Action will also help your family to achieve the same results. You will be an inspiration to many people, especially your kids and your actions will encourage others—including your extended family, friends and colleagues—to follow in your footsteps.

You will have better quality relationships with your family and friends and you will be better at developing new relationships. You will achieve a new level of respect among family, friends and business colleagues and you will feel an increased sense of self-esteem and self-actualization. Your actions will transform your life from where you are today to where you can be in one year, three years, five years or more.

Overall, you will have a much better knowledge and understanding of key health, exercise and nutrition issues. You will have a more positive and proactive mindset about exercise and a new zest for life with unlimited energy. Your confidence will soar, enabling you to achieve new goals and new heights. You will know that you can do things you thought you would never do again.

The choice is yours, but I hope I have convinced you that from now on, you are on a mission with exciting **projects** which you will complete with **energy** and **resolve**. You will find a worthy **cause** and you will get fully **involved** in your new passion. Your new lifestyle mission will be **extraordinary**.

Your New Lifestyle Mission

So now you know! You need to be on a mission if you want to succeed and achieve your dream with the ultimate prize of a long, healthy life with a great quality lifestyle. Improving your health will increase your life expectancy and add many high-quality years to your life. This is an important step for you to take if you need to do something about your life, your health, your weight, the food you eat and especially your fitness level, once and for all.

Your new lifestyle mission has **5 Essential Stages** to ease you into the best shape of your life regardless of your age, weight or current fitness level:

Stage 1—Your Mission Decision
Stage 2—Your Current Fitness Level
Stage 3—Your Project Plan
Stage 4—Your Project Implementation
Stage 5—Your Project Review

In the remaining chapters of Part 3 we will examine the 5 Stages one by one. It is important to remember, however, that these stages are all part of an ongoing process and are very much linked to one other. While you may have a long-term destination in mind, your Mission is the voyage and it will evolve as you develop and grow.

X Your "To Do" List

1. Complete the X Man exercise to help you think about your future journey.
2. Complete the X Factor exercise to see how many of the six elements of R.E.C.I.P.E. you possess.
3. Have you the resolve necessary to change your lifestyle? Ask yourself the two key questions. Where does exercise fit into your priorities and are you prepared to take the time required to adapt to your new lifestyle?
4. Choose exercise that you will enjoy and that you can be passionate about.
5. Find a great cause and get as involved as you can in projects which will be an important part of your new lifestyle.
6. Believe that your new lifestyle mission will be extraordinary.

"Energy and persistence conquer all things."
—Benjamin Franklin

CHAPTER 12

YOUR X FACTOR DECISION

The first stage of your new lifestyle is to consider and then decide what your mission is going to be. In the last chapter we discussed the six key ingredients of the X Factor and it follows that these are also important ingredients for your mission. So before we go any further, I would like you to take some time to review the six ingredients which make up the acronym **RECIPE** and ask yourself the following questions:

R—Resolve
- Are you committed enough to make this happen?
- Where do exercise and your health fit into your priorities?
- Are you prepared to allocate the time required to your new lifestyle mission?
- Are you prepared to create the right environment for success?

E—Energetic

- Are you energetic and enthusiastic about your new lifestyle mission?
- Have you got a physical activity that you enjoy or have enjoyed in the past?
- Can you choose something that you believe you can be passionate about?
- Are you excited and raring to get started?

C—Cause

- Do you have a personal cause that will inspire you to succeed?
- If not, can you find something personal that will keep you seriously motivated?
- Have you got a charity in mind that you would like to help?

I—Involved

- Are you prepared to immerse yourself in your new lifestyle mission?
- Will you get involved with other people, coaches and mentors who can support you and help you achieve your mission?

P—Project

- Can you link your cause to a project that you would like to do?
- Are there any local activities that you could turn into a project?
- Do you have any goals that you can turn into a short- or medium-term project, such as a local road race?

E—Extraordinary

- How high on your list of priorities is your new lifestyle mission?
- Do you feel you have the ingredients in place to produce an extraordinary outcome?

Visualization of Your Mission

Having thought about your new journey and lifestyle by answering the questions above about the six ingredients of Your Mission, it is now time to decide your new lifestyle mission. This is where you need to answer questions such as, "How long would you like to live?" and "What quality of life would you like to have?"

To help you answer these questions, take some time and go to a quiet place, sit down and close your eyes. When you are relaxed, try to visualize where you will be and what you will be doing when you are seventy-five, eighty-five or even a hundred. Can you see your husband, your wife, your partner, your kids or grand-kids, your friends? Think about the exercise you will be doing at that age and the food you will be eating. Think about your body—a fit and healthy body! Think about how good you will look and how much better you will feel!

I am sure you are visualizing an attractive place to be. Now ask yourself what you need to do, from a health and fitness point of view, to maximize the chances that your visualization will become a reality. When you look at yourself today and compare that to where you would like to be, is there a gap? How big is it? How are you going to bridge that gap? Have you got a plan in place to make your visualization a reality?

The key now is to decide what you want your lifestyle mission to be. This should be about your health, your weight, your nutrition and especially about your exercise. You need to produce a mission statement which will incorporate your decisions about each of these elements. These will be personal decisions which are unique to you, but to help you with this process I have produced an illustration below.

Illustration of Your New Lifestyle Mission

Your Future Vision—Health

I will transform my way of life so that I will achieve the following:

1. *Significantly increase my life expectancy. One hundred years of age would be nice but an additional ten years over average life expectancy at age sixty-five, (ninety-two for men and ninety-five for women) is a realistic objective.*

2. *Enjoy a high quality of life, free from chronic illness and injury. In particular, I will really focus on my two current high risk factors, heart disease and type 2 diabetes.*

3. *I will gradually reduce my current weight by twenty-five pounds so that my Body Mass Index (BMI) is no more than 25. This will facilitate the achievement of all my other mission objectives.*

4. *I am going to select an appropriate health cause that I can be passionate about.*

Your Future Vision—Exercise

I will get off the couch and transform my life by getting fit and staying fit with exercise as a key priority for the rest of my life as follows:

1. *I like walking, running, cycling and swimming and I am going to gradually build them into my weekly exercise routine. I will explore how I can get involved with exercise groups in my local community.*

2. *I would like to complete a 5K road race initially but eventually (within the next few years) I would like to do a marathon and after that maybe a triathlon.*

3. *I plan to take my exercise outdoors as much as possible and it will also be a key ingredient of future vacations. I want to get back to taking an annual ski vacation and I would also like to do bike trips in the coming years in Europe and California.*

Your Future Vision—Nutrition

I am going to make some healthy changes to what I eat and drink as soon as possible.

1. *I will have a largely (95%) healthy diet with many more vegetables, fruits, pulses and nuts.*

2. *I will try to eliminate or at least minimize the bad food I eat, including too much fast and processed food and way too much sugar.*

3. *I will also significantly reduce the number of sodas and the amount of coffee that I drink, finding healthier choices such as water, natural whole-food smoothies and green or white tea.*

Your New Lifestyle Mission

It is important to consider your new lifestyle mission as a journey into your long-term future. You need to think strategically when contemplating your mission and you need to think long-term. Put simply, what is the "big picture" for you? What are your longer-term lifestyle objectives?

This could be about your health, your weight, your nutrition or your exercise but it is more likely to be, and should be, about all of these. These will be very personal decisions; you must choose a mission to ensure you can bridge the gap between your wishes or dreams and your actions.

I like to think of longer-term missions which are supported by medium-term projects, which in turn are supported by short-term goals. There has to be a link or connection between what you are doing today, your short-term goals and your medium-term projects, as well as your longer-term mission.

Long-Term Mission
- "Big picture" vision
- Long-term strategic focus
- One- to five-year timeframe
- Focus on your health, exercise, weight, nutrition

Medium-Term Projects
- Consistent with Mission
- Timeframe of three to twelve months
- At least one new project every year
- See Chapter 14: Your Project Plan

Short-Term Goals
- Consistent with Mission and Current Project
- Daily, weekly, monthly goals
- See Chapter 14: Your Project Plan—SMART Goals

While the focus of your mission is longer-term and big picture, it is equally important to live in the present. While you need to think about your future, you also need to focus on the present, the magic of the moment. You have your dreams and many back-to-back projects to complete, but your journey should be the best part, and you must learn to enjoy each day, even when you have to put up with some discomfort or pain.

Back-to-Back Projects

While your mission will be long-term and big picture, you will need to break it down into significant medium-term projects which run back-to-back and which are consistent with your new lifestyle.

The chart below illustrates how you should aim to have progressive back-to-back projects but only one project on the go at a time, especially at the start. If you want to achieve your mission objectives, you need to have a map of how you are going to do it.

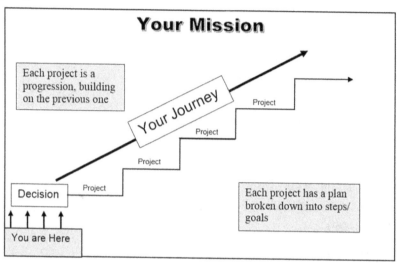

Breaking your mission down into medium-term projects makes this much more achievable and I will return to this subject in Stage 3, which we will discuss in Chapter 14: Your Project Plan. However, before you can decide what your first project will be, you need to take stock of the present in Stage 2, which we will do next in Chapter 13: Your Current Fitness Level.

✗ Your "To Do" List

1. Review the six ingredients which make up the acronym RECIPE and answer the list of questions.
2. Take some time out and go to a quiet place (or go for an easy walk) and do the visualization exercise.
3. Decide what you want your new lifestyle mission to be and record these decisions in your mission statement.
4. Start thinking about your first medium-term project and the short-term goals you will need to put in place to achieve it.

> *"There is no passion to be found playing small—in settling*
> *for a life that is less than the one you are capable of living."*
> **—Nelson Mandela**

CHAPTER 13

YOUR CURRENT FITNESS LEVEL

In Chapter 11, you learned that there are 5 stages to your new lifestyle mission. In the last chapter our focus was on Stage 1—Your X Factor or Mission Decision and so you should now have a much clearer picture of what your future way of life looks like.

As we learned in Stage 1, while the focus of your mission is longer-term, it is equally important—probably even more so—to live in the present, especially at the start. Once you know where you are heading, you have to figure out how you are going to get there. In the next chapter, we will discuss Your Project Plan but before we can do this you must have a very clear understanding of where you are starting from. So Stage 2—Your Current Fitness Level is a critically important step if you want to start your new lifestyle mission in a way which gives you the greatest chance of success.

Your first project must be the right one for you, taking your specific set of circumstances into account. You need to be completely honest with yourself in your appraisal of your current fitness level.

Medical Clearance

It is always a good idea to get the "all clear" from your doctor before you start a new exercise regimen but especially one as important and significant as your new lifestyle mission. I recommend that you discuss your plans with your doctor and seek both his advice and support. I am sure this will be a very worthwhile exercise.

Besides the fitness levels we will discuss shortly, I encourage you to record some key health measures as your starting point or benchmark, from which you can monitor your progress over the coming weeks, months and years. You should consider the following measures:

1. Your Body Mass Index

While this is not a perfect measure (few measures are!), your Body Mass Index (or BMI) is a popular measure and a reliable indicator of your level of body fat. The easiest way to find yours is to Google "BMI calculator" and enter your height and weight into the fields or tables provided. Your score will probably fall into one of these three areas:

Normal: 18.5 - 24.9
Overweight: 25.0 - 29.9
Obese: 30.0 and above

Obviously your goal in the long term should be to get your BMI into the normal range.

2. Your Waist-to-Height Ratio

This is another important measure which is gaining popularity and credibility and should be used in conjunction with your BMI. As we get older, largely because of our diet but also because of the lack of exercise, our waists continue to get bigger and bigger as we accumulate dangerous visceral fat around some of our most important organs. So we need to pay particular attention to this measure because it is correlated with abdominal obesity.

Your waist-to-height ratio is defined as your waist circumference divided by your height and is a measure of the distribution of your body fat. To measure your waist, place a tape measure around your body at the top of your hipbone. This is usually at the level of your belly button. You calculate your waist-to-height ratio as follows:

Waist / Height %
Example: Waist = 34 inches, Height = 68 inches
34/68 = 50%

Your goal should be to have a waist-to-height ratio of less than 53% for men and less than 49% for women. Anything more puts you at greater risk of weight-related health problems as shown in the table below.

Weight	Males	Females
Healthy Weight	43% to 52%	42% to 48%
Overweight	53% to 62%	49% to 57%
Obese	Over 63%	Over 58%

3. Your Waist-to-Hips Ratio

Your waist-to-hips ratio is a third useful measure which you can use in conjunction with your BMI and your waist-to-height ratio. It measures the ratio of the circumference of your waist to that of your hips. You measure your waist as before and your hips at the widest part of your buttocks with the tape measure parallel to the floor. You calculate your waist-to-hips ratio as follows:

Waist / Hips %
Example: Waist = 35 inches, Hips = 40 inches
35/40 = 87.5%

The waist-to-hips ratio is another indicator of your health and the risk of developing serious health conditions. Research shows that people with "apple-shaped" bodies, who have more weight around the waist, face more health risks than those with "pear-shaped" bodies, who have more weight around the hips. This indicator is used as a measurement of obesity which in turn is a possible indicator of other more serious health conditions. You can identify your level of risk in the table below.

Risk Level	Males	Females
Low Risk	95% or Lower	80% or Lower
Moderate Risk	96% to 100%	81% to 85%
High Risk	Over 100%	Over 85%

So in the example above, a waist-to-hips ratio of 87.5% is low risk if you are male but high risk if you are female.

4. Other Key Health Measures

I also encourage you to discuss some other key health measures with your doctor. Each of us will have different measures on which we need to focus but they are likely to include your blood pressure, blood sugar and key cholesterol measures.

Two other important gauges to consider are how much sleep you get and how many hours a day you spend sitting. You should track your nightly sleep for a week or two and see what your average is. Ideally it should be in the seven to nine hour range. An average of less than seven hours per night is not good in the long run.

You read earlier that sitting has become the new smoking. This is undoubtedly a provocative statement but you have been warned! Life in the twenty-first century means that we spend much of our waking time sitting, whether we are at work, at school or at play. The average adult spends *nine hours a day sitting,* which is a lot. Moreover, that is often compounded by little planned exercise as well as precious little unplanned (baseline) exercise. If you are on the wrong side of that average you need to pay particular attention to your baseline activities. You need to get up and out of your chair and move for at least 5 minutes every hour.

If your schedule doesn't allow you to do that, then work around it or—better still—change your schedule if you value your life!

Your Current Exercise

What is your current level of physical activity? What kind of exercise do you do and how many days a week do you do it? How many hours do you exercise and what distance do you cover? At what speed do you go or what is your pace? These are all important questions you need to answer and the table below sets out three examples for aerobic activities—walking, running and swimming.

EXAMPLES	Walking	Running	Swimming
Days per Week	3	2	2
Hours per Week	2	1	1
Distance (in Miles)	4	4	1
Speed (MPH)	2	4	1
Pace (Minutes per Mile)	30	15	60

You should record your weekly exercise in a similar way. As it is likely that it will vary from week to week it usually helps to record what your most and least active weeks look like so that you can extrapolate your average or typical week. In the table below I have set out a sample to help you with this. This does not have to be precise but it should provide a realistic appraisal of what a typical week's exercise looks like for you. Don't forget to include any strength exercises and stretching you are doing.

SAMPLE	Most Active	Least Active	Average
Days per Week	3	1	2
Hours per Week	3	1	2
Distance (in Miles)	6	2	4
Speed (MPH)	2	2	2
Pace (Minutes per Mile)	30	30	30

Your 1 Mile Fitness Challenge

I would like you to complete a one mile fitness challenge, assuming you have clearance from your doctor to do so. The result of this challenge will be the starting point for your first project, which we will discuss in the next chapter. With this benchmark in place, you will be able to monitor your progress from this day forward.

The table below provides two samples as well as room for your results. In sample one, the one mile challenge is covered in twenty minutes, which is a brisk walk at three miles per hour. In sample two the time is faster at fifteen minutes, which is a slow run at four miles per hour.

1 Mile Challenge	Sample 1	Sample 2	Your Results
Description	Brisk Walk	Slow Run	
Time for 1 Mile (Minutes)	20	15	
Speed (MPH)	3	4	
Pace (Minutes per Mile)	20	15	

The best way to take on this challenge is to do it a few times and you can do this over the course of a week or two. You need to find somewhere safe that you can walk or run continuously for one mile. A local track would be a great place to do this as four times around equals one mile. If that is not an option you could measure out a mile in your neighborhood using your vehicle trip meter.

The first time you do the challenge, take it nice and easy. Let's assume you are walking so you start out at a pace that you know you can keep up for a mile. Let's say it takes you twenty-three minutes; you now have a standard you know you can beat.

The second time you do the challenge, push yourself a bit harder so you can feel it in your breathing but it is still comfortable. Let's say it takes you twenty-one and a half minutes this time; this is your new standard. Now the third time is going to be your final challenge. I want you to push yourself harder but I don't want you to put yourself in a stressful position. You should be breathing heavily by the end of this third challenge but you should not get into a state of serious oxygen debt. That is not the purpose of the challenge. You want to find your current fitness level, not your pain threshold.

Let's assume you do the third challenge in twenty minutes and so this becomes your one mile fitness benchmark. What is interesting about the three challenges is that you have already made significant progress from twenty-three minutes to twenty and you did it without having excessively stressed yourself. One of the great things about exercise when you are starting is that you can make this kind of progress quite quickly.

Selecting Your Fitness Level

So now you should have a very good knowledge and understanding of your current level of fitness. To recap, before you start a new exercise regimen, you should discuss your plans with your doctor and you should record some key health measures including your:

- Body Mass Index (BMI)
- Waist-to-Height Ratio
- Waist-to-Hips Ratio
- Other Key Health Measures, including your daily amount of sleep and sitting

You have recorded your current weekly exercise and you have completed the one mile fitness challenge. Armed with this information it is time to select your appropriate starting level from the 5 Progressive Levels of Exercise and the Summary Allocation of Your Exercise Time from Chapter 10 which I have set out below for you convenience. You can also use the summary sheets for each level of 5XFT which are set out at the end of Chapter 10.

Summary Allocation of Your Exercise Time

	Level 1	Level 2	Level 3	Level 4	Level 5
Days/Week	4	5	5	5	6
Hours/Week	3	4	5	6	7
Primary Aerobic Activity	Walk	Walk/ Run	V Slow Run	Slow Run	Run
Aerobic Time	150	210	225	230	240
Strength Time	30	30	45	60	60
High Intensity Time	0	0	30	40	60
Cross-training Time	0	0	0	30	60
Total Time (Minutes)	180	240	300	360	420
Avg. Intensity (METS)	3.3	5.0	6.0	6.7	7.1
Total Energy (MET Mins.)	600	1200	1800	2400	3000

While I have chosen walking and running as the primary aerobic activity in the table above, you could of course choose other activities such as swimming or biking. Let us also use your one mile fitness challenge to help you choose your appropriate level.

Level 1: This is the first level of exercise and is the one for you if you have been inactive for at least three months or you have been doing less than two hours of exercise a week for an extended period. It is likely that you walked your one mile fitness challenge and your time was twenty minutes or more.

At this level your primary aerobic activity is walking and you will work your way gradually up to the recommended minimum exercise level of three hours a week over four days. You should be very comfortable exercising at this level before you consider moving to Level 2.

Level 2: This is the second level of exercise and is the one for you if you are already exercising three hours a week on a regular basis. It is likely that your one mile fitness challenge was a brisk walk and you may have even done some running. Your time was probably under twenty minutes.

At this level you will progress gradually from walking to very slow running up to the recommended level of four hours a week over five days. You should be comfortable exercising at this level before you consider moving to Level 3.

Level 3: This is the third level of exercise and is the one for you if you are already exercising four hours a week on a regular basis. It is likely that you were able to run or jog your one mile fitness challenge and your time was probably around fifteen minutes.

At this level you will progress gradually to the recommended level of five hours a week over five days. You should be very comfortable exercising at this level before you consider moving to Level 4.

Level 4: This is the fourth level of exercise and is the one for you if you are already exercising five hours a week on a regular basis. It is likely that you ran your one mile fitness challenge and your time was probably around thirteen minutes.

At this level you will progress gradually up to the recommended level of six hours a week over five days. You should be very comfortable exercising at this level before you consider moving to Level 5.

Level 5: This is the fifth and final level of exercise and is the one for you if you are already exercising a total of six hours a week on a regular basis. It is very likely that you ran your one mile fitness challenge and your time was probably around twelve minutes.

At this level you will progress gradually up to the recommended level of seven hours a week over six days. You should be very comfortable exercising at this level before you consider moving beyond it.

X Your "To Do" List

1. Get the "all clear" from your doctor before you start a new exercise program.
2. Record your key health measures as discussed in this chapter.
3. Track your weekly activity for a few weeks to establish your current exercise benchmark.
4. Complete the one mile fitness challenge and with this benchmark in place, you will be able to monitor your progress from this day forward.
5. Select your appropriate starting level from the 5 Progressive Levels of Exercise.

"No matter how slow you go, you are
still lapping everybody on the couch!"
—Unknown

CHAPTER 14

YOUR PROJECT PLAN

N ow that you have chosen your new lifestyle mission and you have a good knowledge and understanding of your current fitness level, your next task is to select your first project. Each project has a life of its own and can be broken down into milestones or steps along the way. You will make great progress when there is a clear connection between the repetitive nature and sometimes even drudgery of your short-term goals and your medium-term project objectives.

Focus On One Project at the Start

If you have more than one significant self-improvement project going at a time, you may succeed for a while. However, it is considerably better and easier to focus on just one significant challenge at a time. For example, the willpower required to quit smoking is hard enough without simultaneously taking on other major changes. If you try to quit smoking and lose weight at the same time there is a good chance that you will ultimately fail at both.

Think of your resolve as a tank of fuel which gets depleted when you have too many things going on at the same time. One significant health and fitness project at a time is especially important for folks who have busy work and life schedules. This is why folks who make lists of New Year's resolutions often fail—they have so many balls in the air at the same time that they all end up eventually falling down.

Thus, focusing on a significant new exercise project and a major new weight loss diet at the same time is probably not a good idea; you would have two major projects on which to focus simultaneously. Choosing an exercise project and building in some realistic nutrition and weight loss goals for the duration of the project is a much better way to go.

Your First Project

Of course your first project should be consistent with both your long-term mission and your current level of fitness. It should be substantial enough to last at least three months but certainly no more than twelve. I prefer to focus on a relatively short timeframe for your first project so you can get an early win under your belt and set yourself up for future success.

I am a big fan of choosing a 5K road race (3.1 Miles) for your first exercise project because these races work so well, whether you are just starting out, or if you are getting back into exercise after a period of inactivity. Now you might be thinking that there is no way you will be able to do that! But I promise you—millions of people just like you do them all the time. Don't think of them as races; see them as a fun day out for you and your family and friends to enjoy and celebrate at the end of your project.

As well as being great fun, a 5K race gives you a clear objective to strive for at the end of your first project over three to four months. A target like that also facilitates the "training" you will need to do and helps you tick all the boxes for a successful medium-term project, whether you are walking, running or both.

Your Projects

Every project needs a plan and your plan should always focus on your desired result or outcome. Working backwards from your desired result makes it a lot easier for you to set your project objectives and goals.

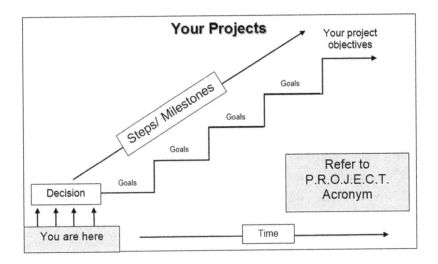

It will also help you if you record your daily actions in a project diary or journal. You are ultimately responsible for project execution and you are more likely to succeed when you review your daily and weekly training on an ongoing basis.

You should always plan to celebrate your success at the end of your project and then plan to take some time out to evaluate your progress and select your next endeavor. To help you remember and apply these important elements to your projects, I have developed another acronym that should be easy for you to remember—P.R.O.J.E.C.T.

P.R.O.J.E.C.T.

P—Plan

R—Results

O—Objectives

J—Journal

E—Execution

C—Celebrate

T—Time Out

The first three—plan, results and objectives—are key elements of your project plan, and we will discuss these in this chapter. The next two, journal and execution, are important elements of your project implementation which we will consider in Chapter 15. The last two, celebrate and time out, are important elements of your project evaluation which we will examine in Chapter 16.

Your Project Plan

Planning for the future is important in most parts of your life. This is true for school, college, work, sport and it is also true for your exercise projects. As the popular saying goes, "If you fail to plan, plan to fail."

Preparation really is half the battle and every project requires a comprehensive plan to be successful. Your plan is a road map of how you are going to get from point A, where you are now, to point B, where you want to be at some point in the future.

I find the best way to develop a plan is to decide on the result or outcome you would like to achieve at point B (the end of your project) and then work backwards to where you are now at point A. Of course, you have to decide how much time you have to allocate to your project but if this project is a high priority in your life, time is unlikely to be a limiting factor.

Your plan should have a timetable with milestones along the way that mark your steps towards the completion of your overall project objectives. I will develop this idea further in the next 2 sections—Project Results and Project Objectives—as these are both integral elements of your plan.

Your plan should incorporate whatever it takes to enable you to achieve your overall objectives including help, support, advice and coaching. Of course, you have to *believe* you can achieve your project objectives, but even if you do, without a plan you are likely to fail and your objectives will just be wishful thinking.

Project Results

It really is very important to think carefully about the results or outcome that you want to achieve for your project. If this is the first project of your new lifestyle mission you want to ensure that the six key ingredients of your mission

RECIPE are effectively cultivated throughout the project. This will set a firm foundation for your mission and future projects.

Just as a reminder—if you haven't got a passion already, you want to give yourself the best chance of developing it by the end of the project. Your resolve to complete your project and achieve your desired results must not waiver. You should ideally get involved with other likeminded people to support you and if you can, add a personal cause to the mix. These are all important dimensions to your project and will give it the last element of "extraordinary" which will greatly enhance your chances of achieving the results you desire.

My Clearwater Project

Over the years I have chosen many projects this way. I have already told you about the London marathon back in 1987, but another favorite of mine is the Clearwater triathlon in Florida in 2002. This was the year before I moved to Mt. Pleasant in South Carolina with my family.

At the end of the summer in 2001, I decided to choose the Clearwater triathlon the following spring as my next project. This would get me through the winter months and give me something to look forward to. I also decided to do two other things to ensure I achieved the outcome I wanted. First, I asked Paul Newman's "Hole in the Wall Gang" if I could race on their behalf and raise money at the same time. They are one of my favorite charities. Second, my family got involved in the project when we decided to have a vacation at Disney after the race. Look out for the best parts of this story in Chapter 15.

Project Illustration

You should choose an appropriate first project, taking your current fitness level and your personal circumstances into account. In this illustration, we will assume that you have decided you want to complete a 5K road race as the primary result for your first project. You are currently exercising three hours a week and you are walking at around three miles per hour, which is a pace of twenty minutes per mile. You would like to increase your intensity and progress to running and you feel that running at least some of your first 5K, if not all of it, is realistic.

You would also like to reduce the amount of junk food you eat, especially French fries and sodas, and you would like to lose some weight as a result of both your improved diet and increased exercise. These would be your secondary desired results.

So let us consider our illustration based on the following guidelines:

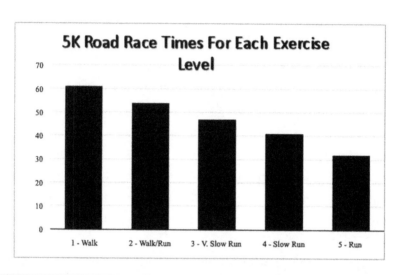

5K Road Race	Level 1	Level 2	Level 3	Level 4	Level 5
Aerobic Exercise	Walk	Walk & Run	Very Slow Run	Slow Run	Run
Projected Time (Mins.)	62	53	47	40	31
Minutes Per Mile	20	17	15	13	10
Miles Per Hour	3.0	3.5	4.0	4.6	6.0

Your Primary Result

For the primary result of your first project, you decide you want to complete a 5K Road Race in fifty minutes. You choose a local race which is thirteen weeks away. If there isn't a local race available then why not take a short vacation or weekend away and choose another race; there are likely to be many choices available.

Your Secondary Results

For your secondary results, you decide you are going to limit your French fries and sodas to one meal a week and as a result of your improved nutrition and exercise you want to lose ten pounds by the end of the project.

Project Objectives

When you have a clear picture of the project results you desire, by working backwards, it is relatively easy to decide on your project objectives. Setting project objectives and goals is really important as they give you clear direction. Having a clear understanding of both where you are going and how you are going to get there significantly increases your chances of a successful outcome.

In the same way that your mission needs to be broken down into projects, your project objectives need to be broken down into smaller steps or milestones along the way, so that you always know you are on track and heading in the right direction.

While your focus, initially at least, should be on one project at a time, it is important that you do not have too many individual project objectives and that these goals are consistent with your overall project plan. It is also important that your goals do not conflict with each other. The more competing demands you face the more time you spend worrying about them. If you have clear, non-conflicting goals you are much more likely to make progress and succeed. If you don't, you are more likely to waste time worrying and you will probably get stuck and fail.

S.M.A.R.T. Goals

Your goals need to be effective, that is they are set up in a way that makes you more likely to achieve them. I have used the goal-setting acronym S.M.A.R.T. for many years, going right back to my days in HR management, over thirty years ago. I have always found it to be very useful, especially when you are just starting out. It is important to remember, though, that goal-setting is just a starting point; without a clear action plan as mentioned above, goals can become nothing more than wishful thinking!

S—Specific

Specific goals are clear and easy to understand. They should not be vague like "I am going to start running" or "I am going to lose weight ". They tell you precisely what you have to do to succeed and how you will know when you achieve them.

Applying the illustration above, a good example of specific goals is:

- My primary objective is to complete the local Susan G Komen Race for the Cure, 5K Run and Walk on October 31.
- My secondary objectives are to limit French fries and sodas to one meal a week and to lose ten pounds by October 31.

M—Measurable

A measurable goal means that you can measure actual performance against a standard so that you know how you are doing throughout the project. So using the illustration above, you can applying a measurable target of fifty minutes to your primary objective as follows:

- My primary objective is to complete the local Susan G Komen Race for the Cure, 5K Run and Walk on October 31, in fifty minutes.

Your secondary objective, one meal a week is already measurable. You could also adjust your weight loss goal to one pound a week and not less than ten pounds by October 31, so that you have a measurable target each week.

A—Accountable

Accountability is crucial if you want to complete your first project and achieve your desired result. Ultimately, you are accountable for your own actions but it usually helps to find someone who will hold you accountable—someone you trust and respect and who will not accept excuses.

After determining your goal, write it down in your journal or diary (see later) and get your "accountability partner" to sign it. This person could be your coach, personal trainer, exercise partner or family member. It is much harder to break a commitment that you have made to someone else.

There is a lot to be said for "public" goal-setting, which really just means telling people what your goals are. By doing this, you are much more likely to succeed—probably because of the fear of shame you might feel if you did not achieve them. In a sense, you feel more accountable for achieving your goals when you involve other people.

I always do this! So for example, when I did the London marathon (1987) or the Clearwater triathlon (2002), I organized my charities and started collecting sponsorship money immediately.

You don't have to go to the same lengths to which I went; simply announcing to your family, friends and work colleagues that you are training for the Susan G Komen 5K Run and Walk on October 31 greatly increases your chances of doing it. You do not want to experience the ignominy of having to tell everyone that you failed!

R—Realistic

A realistic goal is challenging but achievable, taking your personal circumstances into account. Don't set a goal which is too demanding and which you are unlikely to accomplish. When you set unrealistic goals you are more likely to quit, especially if you see quite early on that you are not going to be able to reach your target. You also increase the risk of injury when you put yourself under too much pressure.

Equally, you don't want to set a goal which is too easy to achieve, though it is better to be more conservative than to be too optimistic. Remember—your goal is simply a target you want to achieve and possibly even surpass; it should be challenging and you should be confident that you will achieve it.

So let's look at our illustration above. Is 50 minutes a realistic target?

We know you are currently walking at three miles per hour, which is a twenty minute mile pace. If you were to do the 5K today, you should be able to complete it in sixty-two minutes (3.1 miles x 20 minutes). It would not be a bad idea to go out and see what you can do today. So let's say you do this and your time is a very encouraging sixty minutes, which is around 19:20 minutes per mile.

To achieve your target of fifty minutes you would need to drop ten minutes off your time and improve your pace to close to sixteen minutes per mile. This would mean that you would definitely have to run the full 5K (3.1 miles) at what would be a pretty decent clip, given your current level of fitness. That is a lot to ask in around thirteen weeks. It is not impossible, but it is definitely optimistic. So I would adjust your target as follows:

- My primary objective is to complete the local Susan G Komen Race for the Cure 5K Run and Walk on October 31, in fifty-five minutes.

You still need to reduce your time by five minutes and this is a 17:40 minute per mile pace, which is much more achievable and definitely more realistic. It is still challenging, as you will probably have to run at least some of the race.

So, your target is now fifty-five minutes. You are free to try to beat this target by as much as you can but you are not under any pressure. Anything under fifty-five minutes will mean you are successful and you should agree to this change with your "accountability partner".

T—Timed

Your project objectives should have a clear timetable for completion. This means that along with your overall deadline, your objectives should be broken down into shorter-term steps and milestones along the way which will increase the likelihood of you being able to achieve them.

Let us consider our illustration again, where your primary objective is to complete the 5K road race on October 31 in fifty-five minutes. We also know that as of today, you are able to complete 5K (3.1 miles) in sixty minutes, which is 19:20 minutes per mile, and that you are thirteen weeks away from the race. Your secondary objective is to lose ten pounds by October 31.

The table below sets out your starting position with thirteen weeks to go, with weekly steps or milestones all the way to race day. You can monitor your progress throughout the thirteen-week training period by comparing actual weekly performance to your weekly goals. This implies that you do a 5K (3.1 mile) trial or test each week, which you can do if you want to, although you don't have to do one every week. Also, it is unlikely that your progress will be as even or symmetrical as set out in the table.

Weeks to Go	3.1 Miles (5K)	Time	Pace	Weight Loss
13	Starting Position	60:00	19:20	0
12		59:30	19:11	1
11		59:00	19:02	2
10		58:30	18:52	3
9		58:00	18:43	4
8		57:40	18:36	4
7		57:20	18:29	5
6		57:00	18:23	6
5		56:40	18:17	7
4		56:20	18:10	7
3		56:00	18:04	8
2		55:40	17:58	9
1	Race Objective	55:00	17:44	10

✗ Your "To Do" List

1. Choose your first project over a relatively short timeframe of three or four months and I strongly recommend you consider doing a local 5K road race.

2. Develop your project plan using the acronym P.R.O.J.E.C.T. to help you.

3. Focus on the result or outcome you want to achieve, making sure you cultivate the six ingredients R.E.C.I.P.E. from your new lifestyle mission.

4. Use the project illustration from this chapter to guide you in selecting S.M.A.R.T. goals and milestones along the way.

> *"Smart Goals require Effective Actions which Produce Results."*
> **—Jim Kirwan**

CHAPTER 15

YOUR PROJECT IMPLEMENTATION

introduced you to the acronym P.R.O.J.E.C.T. in the last chapter and we covered the first three elements: P for Plan, R for Results and O for Objectives. In this chapter, called Your Project Implementation, we deal with the next two elements: J for Journal and E for Execution. We will consider the final two: C for Celebrate and T for Time Out in the next chapter.

J—Journal

I am a firm believer in recording your project details in your diary or journal. There are a few ways you can do this; some of you may want to track your details online or on your laptop or PC. I definitely show my age and am unashamedly old fashioned in this regard as I like to write stuff down on paper and keep project journals. Journaling truly is an important part of the process and I don't care how you do it, so long as you do it. In the rest of this section, I will refer to the traditional diary or journal but the principles of recording are the same regardless of the method you use.

You can buy training diaries in most sports stores and sometimes you can even get them free. However, a professional sports journal is not necessary; it is very easy to use a blank copybook and just include the details to which I refer below. The first and most important part of your journal is to record your project plans.

Your Project Plan

This needs to be done at the start and if you have followed the instructions in the last two chapters you should be all set. Just as a reminder, however, your project plan will include the following elements:

Your Mission: This is the big picture of where you are going. You only need to record a short summary so that you are constantly reminded of your mission. Refer to the illustration in Chapter 12.

Your Desired Results: This is a summary description of your first project outcome you hope to achieve. In the illustration used in the last chapter, completion of a 5K road race was your primary result. Limiting French fries and sodas to one meal per week and losing ten pounds by the end of the project were your secondary results.

Your Overall Objectives and Weekly Goals: This takes your desired outcome and turns it into SMART goals with steps and milestones along the way. Using the same illustration, the table at the end of the previous chapter sets out your starting position with thirteen weeks to go. Weekly steps or milestones are then recorded, all the way to race day. This allows you to monitor your progress throughout the thirteen-week training period by comparing actual weekly performance to your weekly goals.

Your Training Program: You need to follow an appropriate training program which takes your current level of fitness into account and which will enable you to turn your goals into results. This is an important part of your Project Plan which should be recorded in your journal. Using our illustration from above, I have produced a sample 5K Road Race Training Program Summary for thirteen weeks, based on exercising five days a week. You should follow a similar approach in your personal training program.

SAMPLE: 5K Road Race—13 Week Training Program Summary

Weeks To Go	Day 1	Day 2	Day 3	Day 4	Day 5
13	Walk 40 Pace 20:00	Walk 30 ST 15	Walk 40 Pace 20:00	Walk 30 ST 15	Walk 40 Pace 19:20
12	Walk 40 Pace 19:30	Walk 30 ST 15	Walk 40 Pace 19:40	Walk 30 ST 15	Walk 45 Pace 19:11
11	Walk 40 Pace 19:20	Walk 30 ST 15	Walk 40 Pace 19:30	Walk 30 ST 15	Walk 50 Pace 19:02
10	Walk 40 Pace 19:10	Walk 30 ST 15	Walk 40 Pace 19:20	Walk 30 ST 15	Walk 55 Pace 18:52
9	Walk 40 Pace 19:00	Walk 30 ST 15	Walk 40 Pace 19:10	Walk 30 ST 15	Walk 55 Pace 18:43
8	Walk 45 Pace 18:55	Walk 30 ST 15	Walk 40 Pace 19:00	Walk 30 ST 15	Walk 60 Pace 18:36
7	Walk 45 Pace 18:45	Walk 30 ST 15	Walk 45 Pace 18:55	Walk 30 ST 15	Walk 60 Pace 18:29
6	Walk 45 Pace 18:40	Walk 30 ST 15	Walk 45 Pace 18:50	Walk 30 ST 15	Walk 60 Pace 18:23
5	Walk 45 Pace 18:35	Walk 30 ST 15	Walk 45 Pace 18:45	Walk 30 ST 15	Walk 60 Pace 18:17
4	Walk 45 Pace 18:30	Walk 30 ST 15	Walk 45 Pace 18:40	Walk 30 ST 15	Walk 60 Pace 18:10
3	Walk 45 Pace 18:25	Walk 30 ST 15	Walk 45 Pace 18:35	Walk 30 ST 15	Walk 60 Pace 18:04
2	Walk 45 Pace 18:20	Walk 30 ST 15	Walk 45 Pace 18:30	Walk 30 ST 15	Walk 60 Pace 17:58
1	Walk 40 Pace 18:20	Walk 30 ST 15	Walk 30 Pace 20:00	Rest	**5K Race Pace 17:44**

Important Notes:
- Walk 40 = Walk for Forty Minutes
- Pace 20:00 = Twenty Minutes per Mile
- ST 15 = Strength Training for 15 Minutes

You should record your actual daily activity and whichever way you decide to do this, make sure you give yourself plenty of space. That is why using a simple blank copybook is great; you can give yourself all the space you need to record what you want to record.

Your Daily Activity

You should record the following information each day:

- Time, day and date (e.g. 6:00pm, Wednesday, 26 February)
- Your actual time spent walking and running, including warm up and cool down
- Your actual time spent doing strength and stretching exercises
- Your total time spent exercising
- Your speed in miles per hour or your pace in minutes per mile
- Your distance in miles, broken down into warm-up, main workout and cool down
- Did you achieve your goal for the day, the week?
- How did your weekly 5K trial (3.1 miles) go compared to your target?
- Notes about your day, including things like how you felt at the start, after your warm-up, during your main workout and at the end. Did you drink enough water?
- You could even record notes about the weather, the temperature and your mood
- Make sure you also record your weight in your journal. There are different schools of thought on how often you should weigh yourself. I like to do this at the same time each day and I usually weigh myself just before I get into the shower after training. By doing this you can keep a close eye on how you are progressing compared to your goal. Of course,

you will notice some fluctuations in your weight when you do it this way but it will keep you accountable and motivated to achieve your goal.

All this recording of information in your journal may seem like a lot of work to you now, but it is all part of the process of reinforcing your new lifestyle. After a few weeks of recording what you do, you will start to learn a lot about yourself and you will see the great progress you are making each week.

I regularly make direct comparisons between two or more workouts that are a few weeks apart, to see how I am progressing and it is highly motivating to see that my average speed has dropped by a few seconds. If you decide to do the weekly trial as part of your training program, this will be a great source of motivation as you will make continuous progress—I promise!

E—Execution

Project execution is about putting the plan which you have recorded in your journal into action. Of course it is much easier said than done! Nevertheless, as I said earlier, preparation is half the battle; if you have a sound project plan focused on results with S.M.A.R.T. goals and a realistic training program, you are much more likely to succeed with the not-so-simple matter of executing your project. As project execution is a broad term, I have broken it down under the following headings:

- Show up
- Think positive
- Effort is rewarded
- Ongoing review
- Do this with others
- Use charity sponsorship

Show Up

It may sound ridiculously obvious as you read this but in my experience showing up, or not showing up, as the case may be, is the principal reason why folks either succeed or fail to achieve their goals. The greatest risk exists at the start and unfortunately this is where so many folks fall by the wayside. If you fail to achieve your short-term goals, then as sure as night follows day, you will fail with both your medium-term projects and ultimately your longer-term mission.

I see this happen all the time. Let me illustrate with a specific example in the pie chart below.

■ No Show ▨ Once or Twice ▨ Occasionally ▨ All the Time

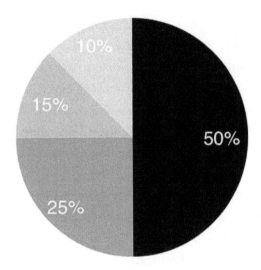

When we started a new walk and run club in Mount Pleasant, my home town, some five hundred members signed up initially. Of these, about half never showed up even once. Of the two hundred fifty who did show up, only about half of these returned. Of the remaining members, some of these showed up only occasionally but only about fifty showed up all the time. So that's one out of every ten who signed up got into the habit of showing up.

Now, every one of the fifty regulars are on a mission and are making incredible strides forward with their health and fitness. From the couch in many cases, they started walking and running, slowly building up their fitness and collectively losing a lot of weight. They showed up early in the morning, after work and on weekends and got into the good habit of exercising with a group of likeminded folks. They are now running half marathons and marathons and completing triathlons and trail runs. I am sure they won't mind me describing them as average, everyday folks who simply made the decision to get fit and stay healthy and then implemented their plans. They have made some great friends and have built a new social life around their new lifestyle mission.

You have to take action to achieve your project goals and you can get started by simply showing up. The key takeaway here is: *if you just show up, amazing things will happen!*

Think Positive

Your initial reaction to my suggestion that you try to do a 5K road race may have been something like, "Over my dead body!" but I am sure you are warming to the idea by now. Millions of people complete road races every year—young, old and everyone in between. Some walk, some run and many do a bit of both; regardless of how they do it, the key thing is that they do it. And as a bonus, they end up having a lot of fun along the way! If you keep reminding yourself about the result you want to achieve, you will get through the difficult days, especially at the start.

I could count on one hand the number of times I feel bad after exercising. Sure, I sometimes feel tired and often a bit sore but I am nearly always glad that I did it. It is hard to beat the feeling of triumph you have when you accomplish your training goal for the day and you will nearly always hear your training buddies say the same thing, too. You will often see group members slapping each other on the back or doing high fives at the end of a long or hard training session.

It is very easy to have a negative mindset about exercise. Unfortunately, at a time when comfort and convenience are cherished more than ever before, exercise is often perceived as a chore—something to get out of the way as quickly as possible. If you are one of the people who currently thinks negatively about exercise, you will have to take a leap of faith and try to switch to positive mode. I hope this book will help you do just that.

Ultimately, exercise will have to be a high priority in your life and you will have to see it as fun and enjoyable if you want to sustain this positive mindset. However, you have to start somewhere! Knowing that you will feel great afterwards will help you make that necessary leap of faith. So, if you are lying in bed on a cold, dark morning debating with yourself about whether to get up and exercise or roll over and go back to sleep, think positive! Visualize how great you will feel when you are finished and *get out of bed!*

Effort is Rewarded

The first ingredient of the X Factor is **resolve** and you certainly need that to sustain your efforts each day, especially at the start. The second ingredient is **energetic** and there is no getting away from the fact that you will need to work hard if you want to succeed. No one said this would be easy, but *you can do this* if you persevere and maintain your energy and enthusiasm on an ongoing basis. You will fall off the horse from time to time, we all do, but if you can just put it behind you and keep trying, you will get there eventually.

What I love about the exercise we are talking about is that anyone can do it! There is no talent required but effort and hard work are rewarded. Once you start, you will see your progress almost immediately and that progress will continue if you just keep trying. I have seen folks starting out at a pace of twenty-minute miles go to fifteen minutes within a few months and then they continue to achieve significant improvements as their pace falls to ten-minute miles. Of course, your rate of progression will be directly related to the effort you put in. One other thing to be aware of, by the way, is that once you reach that ten-minute mile pace, your progress from that point on will definitely be in much smaller chunks of time.

There is a famous quote which says, "The harder I work, the easier it gets" or another version which says, "The harder I work, the luckier I get". Whichever way you say it, both are highly relevant to exercise, particularly aerobic activities such as running, swimming, cycling, rowing, skiing, etc.

Ongoing Review

By using your journal to record your Project Plan and your Daily Activity you are nicely set up to review your progress on an ongoing basis. Your plans include your SMART Goals with weekly steps and milestones, so by tracking your daily exercise you can monitor how you are doing against your overall plans on an ongoing basis. As your project unfolds you will know if you are on track, ahead of or behind schedule and you will be able to make appropriate adjustments to increase the chances of achieving your project objectives.

Weeks To Go	Days/Week	Hours/Week	Goal Pace	Actual Pace
13	5	3:30	19:20	19:05
10	5	3:45	18:52	18:50
7	5	4:00	18:29	18:40
4	5	4:00	18:10	18:30
1	5	4:00	17:44	17:58

If you are on track or ahead of schedule, you certainly don't need to make any adjustments. If you are behind schedule, as in the illustration above, you will probably know what caused it. It could be that your daily activity has fallen behind or maybe your goal was too optimistic. If you can take actions to get back on track, great! But remember—it is important to make appropriate adjustments considering your current circumstances. In the example above, you fell a little behind but it is not the end of the world. Keep in mind that this is not a workplace appraisal. Things happen, but you want to maintain a positive mindset that will set you up for future success. The outcome in the chart above is still great progress!

Do This With Others

Getting involved with others is one of the six key ingredients of the X Factor and this element is so important that it is worth repeating here. If you implement your project with other people, you will significantly increase your chances of success.

When interviewed during and after *The Biggest Loser*, the competitors inevitably say that they could never have succeeded without the involvement of the competition. Equally, the Healthy Charleston Challenge participants—to a man and woman—all freely admit that they could never have succeeded if they had not gotten involved with the Challenge. The fifty regulars in the Walk and Run Club say exactly the same thing about their involvement with the Club.

It is certainly possible to go it alone but it is much harder; this is especially true for beginners or folks who have been inactive for quite a while. Now don't get me wrong here, you can do this by yourself and some folks are better suited for that than others. However, all other things being equal, it is a lot easier to do this with others. Having said that, I would prefer to see you do this alone than not do it at all. So if, for whatever reason, you have to exercise alone then please go ahead and do it. I have personally done this on many occasions, usually for business reasons, and was successful. If you go this route, however, make sure you implement some of the other suggestions listed below such as sponsorship and reward. Furthermore, if you can, involve your family.

There are many ways for you to plan to exercise with others or get support from others including the following:

- **Existing Group:** The easiest way to do this with others is to join a group that is already doing what you wish to do. This could be in your local community or with work colleagues or friends. You just need to make sure that they share the same aspirations as you now do.

- **Family/Friends:** One way or another you need to get support from your family, your wife, your husband, your partner, even the kids. So why not get them directly involved in the process and you will probably inspire them to follow you.

- **Local Gym:** You could join a local gym or fitness center and participate in any number of group classes from spinning to swimming; this way you are likely to get to know many new people over time. Even if you do not become great friends, the discipline of showing up at the gym with other likeminded folks is half the battle.

- **Run Club/Group:** If you have the option to join a good running group or club, then I strongly recommend that you do so. Most specialty running stores have walking and running groups and they will usually be organized and led by experienced runners who know what they are doing. Make sure you do your research and check that beginners are welcome. They may say you are, but the real test will be how they look after you when you attend for the first time.

- **Training Programs:** Another great approach is to get involved in an organized training program which is appropriate for your current fitness level. Let us assume that your first project will be a 5K road race consistent with the illustration we used in the last chapter. This makes you search for a program that will appropriately train you for a 5K race. I encourage you to check out my training programs, *5X Fitness Transformation* and *Anyone Can Run*.

- **Coach/Trainer:** Another valid approach is to hire a coach or trainer, someone who believes in you and your dream. A good one will help you plan your projects and set realistic goals as well as make sure you stay on track and motivate you to keep going when times get tough. Ultimately, it is up to you to make this happen and you have to do all the hard work but a good coach will be there to support you and hold you accountable along the way. The most successful people, whether it is in business, entertainment, sport or just completing their first project on the road to their new lifestyle mission have coaches to guide them in overcoming obstacles and help them achieve their goals.

- **Role Models:** Surround yourself with people who think like you and are already doing what you want to do. Hang out, ask questions and copy them. Remember, they were exactly where you are now only a short time ago! They will be delighted to help and inspire you and if by some chance they are not, then it is they who have the problem, not you! Think about club members, team members, group members and training program members. Choosing a 5K road race is a great way to get local support and find some role models.

Use Charity Sponsorship

The third of the six key requirements of the X Factor is to develop a **cause**. A great way to do this is to pick an appropriate charity, consistent with your personal cause; the charity may even become your cause! Contact the charity, tell them about your project and ask them if you could raise money for them. They will undoubtedly be delighted to work with you. Your sponsorship of their charity gives you a great way to get actively involved with your project, support a great cause and, at the same time, do something extraordinary to benefit others.

This idea works really well when you are starting out on your new lifestyle mission, as your friends and colleagues will usually be very happy to support you. Over the course of a few years, contributions can wear a bit thin if you keep coming back to the same folks but you can always take a break from your charity and/or try a different one.

I used to do this all the time and my charity of choice was originally the Irish Heart Foundation, then the British Heart Foundation when I lived in London and later Paul Newman's Hole in the Wall Gang.

My Clearwater Story Continued

Let me tell you the rest of my Clearwater triathlon story. As you know, I was still living in Ireland and around September of 2001, I decided to do a triathlon in Clearwater, Florida in April 2002. As that was my next project, I contacted the Hole in the Wall Gang in Ireland and they were delighted that I wanted to raise funds for them. I sent a letter to all my friends, work colleagues and clients asking them to sponsor me and I raised some $13,000; most of my sponsors actually sent a check long before I left for Florida.

I am sure you can see how having this sponsorship in place really focused my mind on the completion of my project. So after seven months of winter training, I was ready and I left Dublin for Clearwater about a week before the race. This was an amazing race for me; it doubled as the Pan American championship, so there were participants from all across the world.

Within thirty seconds of starting the first leg of the triathlon, which was a 1500 meter swim, another participant accidentally kicked me in the face and dislodged my goggles. I wore contact lenses at the time and so this was a mini disaster for me. Did you ever try to put goggles back on in deep water with hundreds of fellow participants swimming by? I struggled for what seemed like a long time and was so upset that I considered throwing in the towel. However, with $13,000 on the line, I told myself to stay calm and I eventually got the goggles back on, though I did have to swim the race with one eye closed, as water kept coming in. Once I got out of the water, I was like a man possessed and even though I finished closer to the back of the race than the front, I passed many on my way to the finish line.

When I got back to Dublin after our vacation in Disney, I very proudly presented my check to the Hole in the Wall Gang. Oh—one last thing. I had Lasik surgery in both eyes within two weeks.

✗ Your "To Do" List

1. I don't care how you do it, so long as you record or journal your projects, starting with your project plans.

2. Choose an appropriate training program for your project and remember, I recommend that you start with a 5K road race.

3. If you want to achieve your project objectives, I recommend that you use as many of the ideas presented in this chapter as you can, from positive thinking to using charity sponsorship.

> *"Insanity: doing the same thing over and over again*
> *and expecting different results."*
> **—Albert Einstein**

CHAPTER 16

YOUR PROJECT REVIEW

n Chapter 14 we covered the first three elements of the P.R.O.J.E.C.T. acronym, P for Plan, R for Results and O for Objectives. In Chapter 15 we discussed J for Journal and E for Execution. So in this chapter we will consider the final two, C for Celebrate and T for Time Out.

C—Celebrate

After all the hard work you put in to get to this point, it is vitally important to celebrate your success. Not only will you enjoy the celebrations but they will reinforce the actions you have taken and you will most likely want to do it all over again.

Road Race Celebrations

Millions of people complete road races every year and have a lot of fun along the way. I will use my local area of Charleston and Mount Pleasant to illustrate what I mean. There are many races to choose from all year long, though the majority take place from October through April, mainly because the summer months are hot. I have chosen four of the most popular races:

- **Susan G. Komen Race for the Cure**: This 5K probably needs no introduction and gets bigger every year. Over ten thousand people participate each year and while this is a race, I believe a celebration of life is a more accurate description of this event. What a great way to start your new lifestyle mission—by celebrating after completing the Susan G. Komen Race for the Cure!
- **Turkey Trot:** This 5K is held each year on Thanksgiving in downtown Charleston and is a very popular family occasion with some eight thousand participants. Many folks start their Thanksgiving festivities by doing this race, often with their extended family. They do the race together and then celebrate together. Another great benefit of doing this race is that you won't feel as guilty from overeating the rest of the day!
- **Reindeer Run:** This 5K really kicks off the festive season in Charleston and is another great family event. It is always held on a Saturday morning at the start of December and downtown Charleston is closed to traffic. It is probably the most child-friendly race I know, with some amazing trophies for all age groups and boy, does everyone celebrate afterwards!
- **Cooper River Bridge Run:** This is one of the biggest 10K road races held anywhere in the world; it averages around forty thousand participants every year. Charleston is not a big town, so this is probably the biggest race per capita of any race anywhere. People come from far and wide to participate and this weekend is probably the number one social event on the local calendar. If you have never been to Charleston, what a great way to celebrate your success after completing your first 10K. By the way, if you do your first 5K in the fall, completing your first 10K the following spring is a realistic target.

So if you haven't done so already, go and check your local area and see what road races exist on your door step. Remember that anyone can participate in these events; you just have to register and pay your entry fee. While there will usually be a competitive element at the front of each race, the vast majority of people participate just for fun and to enjoy the pre- and post-race entertainment. You do not have to win a race to be a winner or to celebrate!

Let me issue a quiet word of warning here. I know many people who said they would never participate—let alone compete—in a road race. However, after completing their first one, they have come back again and again. Somehow they are transformed by the experience and now talk about achieving a personal record. In fact, in some cases they are even challenging for age group awards. Surprisingly, this seems to apply even more, the older folks get!

The bottom line here is that road races are great projects to take on board if you are serious about your health and fitness. The sense of achievement will give you plenty of cause to celebrate. You can start short and easy and progress to long and hard if you want to. There is no shortage of new challenges; you can compete with others or just yourself. It is all up to you.

Celebrate with Rewards

I am also a big fan of celebrating your success by using rewards to help you get across the finish line. I have already described how I have used family trips or vacations as a huge incentive at the end of a project. The celebrations usually start long before the race begins. I have taken my family to Italy, Portugal, Malta, London and Florida on vacations which corresponded to my participation in a triathlon.

You don't have to do what I do, but I can tell you from firsthand experience that this method works very well. It is a great way to ensure you get support from your family for your project, from start to finish. Don't underestimate the importance of family support, especially when they are there to celebrate your success with you at the end!

You can and should also use smaller short-term rewards to celebrate the achievement of your short-term steps and milestones along the way. It could be something as simple as an ice cream, a few beers or a glass of wine or it could be more substantial like going out for dinner. Whatever it is, you should celebrate your ongoing success by linking rewards to the completion of short-term goals.

T—Time Out

At the end of your first project you need to take some time out to review and evaluate your results and consider your options before you decide on your next project. Be careful not to let the euphoria you will feel from your achievement and the race day celebrations cloud your judgment. I have seen many folks jump right into their next project, usually another road race, before they even give themselves a chance to catch their breath.

Give yourself a break for a week or two to recharge your batteries. You will probably find it hard to completely break away from your newfound love, so of course go out for an easy walk or run. However, don't push yourself too hard during this time; at the end of your break I want you to be raring to go!

Evaluation of Your First Project

This should not be too big a deal but you do want to take the time to review how you got on. Assuming you completed your first 5K road race, did it go according to plan? Was your time faster or slower than your race objective? With the benefit of hindsight, was your objective time realistic, too optimistic or too pessimistic? Whatever the answer, ask yourself why. Did you complete your training program with ease or were you under time pressure? Are you suffering from any injuries, no matter how small you feel they may be? What would you do differently next time around?

These are all important questions you need to consider and answer before you jump into your next project. By reflecting carefully on these issues you are much more likely to choose an appropriate project, as you continue the voyage of discovery that is your new lifestyle mission.

Your Next Project

Having completed your first 5K road race (or whatever other project you chose), it is likely that you will want to do another one and you are probably wondering if you should even possibly do something bigger or better. This is an important issue to consider because you can go either way. Most tend to go *bigger* when *better* may be a more appropriate choice.

You should always choose your next project by taking your latest fitness level into account. In the table below, I have produced my guidelines for which of the four most popular road race distances you should do, based on my 5 Progressive Levels of Exercise.

Exercise Level	Exercise Type	5K	10K	Half Marathon	Marathon
1	Walk	Yes	No	No	No
2	Walk/Run	Yes	Yes	No	No
3	Run	Yes	Yes	No	No
4	Run	Yes	Yes	Yes	Maybe
5	Run	Yes	Yes	Yes	Yes

So if you are at the top of Level 1 when completing your first project, it makes sense to progress to Level 2. If you follow the above guidelines, you should choose one of the two shorter race distances. This means you should do either another 5K or perhaps a 10K but definitely not a half marathon or marathon. Your decision will be based on the timing of the races as well, because if you decide to do the longer 10K race you will need more time to prepare. I always recommend doing a 5K as part of your preparation for a 10K anyway.

Having just completed a 5K, you could theoretically do another within a couple of weeks and I would certainly not discourage you from doing that. However, your next project should really give you enough time to work on your speed and intensity. If you walked your first 5K, you should aim to run your second. If you ran the first one, you should focus on increasing your speed.

As with most things in life, focusing on quality over quantity will be beneficial in the longer term; remember—you have plenty of time to do the longer races. Your journey has only started and you want to be ready for each step along the way. So if you decide to do another 5K, give yourself at least two months of training time so that you can focus on improving your speed. If you choose a 10K, you will need at least three months (preferably four) to prepare and you should try to do a 5K race about six weeks before the 10K.

Marathon Mania

The last marathon I did was back in 1988 and there is a reason for that. I thoroughly enjoyed the buzz in training for these races and I am so glad I did them, but they do take their toll on your body. I have some minor lower back issues from my rugby-playing days and so after my fourth marathon, I decided that continuing to train for that distance would not be good for my back and I called it quits.

If you are thinking that you would like to run a marathon, then I strongly encourage you to give it a shot. However, make sure you take it one step at a time and don't do one until you are ready to do it. Take things conservatively, learn to run, focus on quality and give yourself enough time to work your way through the 5 Progressive Levels of Exercise. Make sure you do a 10K before you do a half marathon and then do a half marathon before you do a marathon. Take time out to evaluate each project at its completion before you move on to the next one.

If you approach your projects this way, you are much more likely to succeed, and perhaps more importantly, you are much more likely to avoid injury. As I have said before, the tortoise often triumphs over the hare in the long run.

Runner or Jogger

As a runner for nearly forty years, I undoubtedly have a bias in favor of running or what some folks like to call jogging. Dr. George Sheehan, cardiologist, pioneer of running in the United States and author of the bestselling book *Running and Being: The Total Experience* (one of the first books I read about running) famously said that the difference between a jogger and a runner is an entry blank. On this one point, I respectfully disagree with Dr. Sheehan.

Back in 1984 when I was preparing for my first marathon (The Dublin City Marathon), a work colleague who saw me in my running gear one day asked me what I was doing. When I told him that I was training for the marathon, he replied, "Ah, you're a jogger!" I thought for a moment and responded, somewhat defensively, "No, I'm a runner; I am running as hard as I can go!"

So to be true to myself and my response all those years ago, I always use the term runner and I hate the term jogger. To me, jogging is going out for an intentionally very easy run (i.e. a jog), which is good to do from time to time and great fun when done with a group. On the other hand, running—especially at the start—is not always easy, so we will call it running.

✗ Your "To Do" List

1. After all your hard work, make sure you celebrate your success at the end of your project.
2. Use both short-term and long-term rewards and incentives to help you achieve your goals.
3. Take some time out at the end of your project and evaluate your results before you decide on your next project.
4. Refer to my guidelines above to help you choose your next project and remember that you have plenty of time on your new lifestyle mission.

"The finish line is just the beginning of a whole new race."
—Unknown

PART 4

A FOUNTAIN OF KNOWLEDGE
FOR YOUR NEW LIFESTYLE

INTRODUCTION TO PART 4

If you remember back in Part 1, I introduced you to the 4 Key Drivers of Success. In Part 2 the focus was on **Exercise** and in Part 3 it was on the **X Factor**. In Part 4, I will introduce you to the two remaining key drivers of success: **Knowledge** and **Nutrition**. These are the four key ingredients on which you need to focus if you want to succeed and have a long, happy, high quality life.

Knowledge

When I refer to knowledge, I am referring to knowledge about the other ingredients but especially about your health. Chapter 17 focuses on your health and in Chapter 18, called "Mind Your Brain", I provide some very important information about your brain.

Nutrition

You need to have a good knowledge of nutrition and you should continue to educate yourself and implement healthy eating and drinking initiatives on an ongoing basis. If you could introduce better food and significantly cut the junk from your diet, you would be well on your way to success. Chapter 19 deals with nutrition.

Last Two Chapters

There are two other chapters in Part 4, which provide you with important knowledge about exercise. In Chapter 20, I set out five easy steps to help you to start exercising and finally in Chapter 21, called "Anyone Can Run", I could not resist the temptation to include a chapter about my favorite pastime, running.

CHAPTER 17

KNOWLEDGE—YOUR THIRD KEY DRIVER

L et's talk about knowledge, the third key driver of success, with a focus on your health. While your health is a very important subject to you and your family, I believe we have the tendency to sweep it under the carpet—at least I know I do. We tend to take our health for granted and we really don't like talking about it very much until we have to because we are sick or injured.

The education system does not prioritize health so our general knowledge is actually very limited. Consequently, like many other things in life, including exercise and nutrition, we are left to figure things out for ourselves. We are definitely the most entertained people in the world but probably the least informed. I believe the majority of Americans need a better understanding and knowledge of their health and the extent of the problems we are facing.

In Chapter 1, I referred to four major health problems facing America: obesity, diabetes, Alzheimer's and inactivity. We have already discussed the Inactivity Epidemic and we will discuss Alzheimer's in the next chapter (which is entitled, "Mind Your Brain"). So let's take a look at obesity and diabetes, which are very close cousins and are often referred to as the "Diabesity" epidemic.

Obesity and Diabetes

You are probably fed up with hearing about obesity and diabetes but the numbers involved are so staggering that I feel I need to refer to them here. Some 70% of all Americans are overweight, with a BMI (Body Mass Index) of 25 or more. Of these, about half can be classified as obese, which means they have a BMI of 30 or more. Close to *thirty million* people have type 2 diabetes and about a quarter of these don't even know that they have it. The most staggering figure of all is that over *eighty million* Americans are pre-diabetic.. I think you can see why it is called the diabesity epidemic; this is a scandal of epic proportions!

This is why knowledge is one of my four key drivers; it is our best weapon in fighting the scandal. To illustrate the extent of the knowledge deficit out there let me refer to a childhood obesity quiz from *The Biggest Loser* in 2013. The participants were asked the following five questions:

Question 1: According to the CDC (Centers for Disease Control and Prevention), what percentage of American children aged two to nineteen are obese?

    a.   5%
    b.   12%
    c.   17%
    d.   39%

The correct answer is 17% which, when you think about it, is very high. Nearly one in every five kids are obese compared to my perception of around one or maybe two in a hundred when I was growing up in Ireland back in the sixties and early seventies. This is a huge negative development.

Question 2: What percentage of overweight kids, ages five to ten, already have at least one risk factor for heart disease?

    a.   10%
    b.   25%
    c.   45%
    d.   60%

One team answered A, one answered B and two answered C. What do you think? The correct answer is 60%. Think about that—60% of overweight kids between the ages of five and ten have at least one risk factor for heart disease—are you kidding me? But if you consider the links between overweight and heart disease, it should not really surprise you.

Question 3: According to the CDC, what is the biggest single source of added sugar in children's diets?

    a.   Chocolate
    b.   Fried Foods
    c.   Sugar-Sweetened Drinks
    d.   Ice Cream

The correct answer is the sugar-sweetened drinks but it is fair to say that all four pack a powerful punch and help explain the earlier numbers.

Question 4: Compete this sentence—over the past three decades the childhood obesity rate in America has _____:

    a.   Decreased
    b.   Doubled
    c.   Tripled
    d.   Stayed the Same

All three teams got the correct answer (C), so no marks for getting the right answer here.

Question 5: What percentage of parents of obese kids think their child is either normal or underweight?

    a.   20%
    b.   38%
    c.   51%
    d.   75%

To me, this one is the most shocking of all. The correct answer is 75%. Think about that—three out of every four parents of obese kids think their child is either normal or even underweight! How can this be? If they were asked to choose between overweight and normal, I could understand, but how could a parent think their obese kid is *under*weight? Clearly this is a huge problem and we have much work to do.

Celebrity Apprentice

In another popular television show, *Celebrity Apprentice*, after winning one of the early rounds, participant Lil Jon presented a check to the Diabetes Association. In his summation he said, "Hopefully we can find a cure for diabetes." Now he may have been referring to type 1 diabetes (his mother had that all her life) but is he aware that there is a cure for type 2 diabetes? To be honest, I don't blame Lil Jon, but what about the producers? They let that one get away!

The message here is clear; the numbers demonstrate that we have serious problems that we are not doing enough about. I believe they also demonstrate that the folks do not really understand the true extent of the problems. If people had good knowledge about such important health issues as diabetes, they would be much more likely to make good, informed decisions. So let's take some time to consider type 2 diabetes.

Type 2 Diabetes

It is an absolute scandal that a third of the American population is afflicted by a disease that is 100% reversible through diet and exercise. With the numbers increasing all the time it is clear, to me at least, that drugs are not a viable long-term solution.

Diabetes on its own is the seventh leading cause of death in America but that statistic is very misleading. Diabetes is actually a key element in most of the causes ranked above it, including heart disease, stroke and Alzheimer's. Overall, if you have diabetes your risk of death is about two times higher than your risk without it. Not only that, but you should also consider that your medical expenses will be more than twice as high.

Type 2 diabetes now accounts for some 95% of all diagnosed cases of diabetes. It usually begins with insulin resistance, a disorder in which your cells become resistant to the amount of insulin in your blood. As your blood sugar increases, the body's need for insulin increases but gradually over time your cells become resistant to the effects of the insulin. A high insulin level is the first sign of insulin resistance and the higher your level the worse your insulin resistance. When you reach this point you have type 2 diabetes.

Type 2 diabetes is caused by eating too much bad food and exercising too little. You can eat anything occasionally and get away with it, especially if you are exercising on a regular basis. What you cannot do is eat bad food all the time. Unfortunately, too many of us do just that and it makes us sick and ultimately kills us. Far too much of the standard American diet, which, when abbreviated spells SAD, is bad food. It is largely made up of processed foods with way too much sugar and too many trans-fats. We also consume an excessive amount of saturated fat from meat and dairy products.

In a healthy body with a normal blood sugar level, the pancreas produces insulin in response to sugar in the bloodstream, with glucose taken up by the muscles for energy. If there is excess sugar it gets converted to fat and is stored in your fat cells with much of it stored as belly fat. When visceral fat accumulates around your tummy, it is a major health warning because it leads to inflammation and it targets vital organs including the liver, pancreas and kidneys, where it can do the most harm.

Your blood fat also goes up when you eat too much fat, especially trans-fats from fried foods or saturated fat from meat and dairy. Just like the sugar, if there is excess fat it is stored for future use, which is helpful when food is scarce (which for most of us in America is never) but harmful when it is not. The potential for fat storage in our bodies is huge and unfortunately many folks don't understand the effect these excess sugars and fats have on their weight and health.

Pre-Diabetes

There is no such thing as a "mild" case of type 2 diabetes, nor is there such a thing as "mildly elevated" blood sugar. Anything above normal has a negative effect in your body. As mentioned earlier, nearly thirty million Americans have type 2 diabetes. However, over eighty million have pre-diabetes and as a result are on the path to the full blown variety. If you have diabetes, your average life expectancy is about fifteen years less than people without it. Moreover, it can cripple you long before it kills you.

The Solution

I know it is a lot easier said than done but the solution should be fairly obvious. You clearly need to change the balance of the way you do things. First, you need to reduce or stop doing some things and then you need to start or do more of some others. Let's start with the things you need to stop doing or do less of.

You should avoid or at least minimize the foods with too much sugar and fat from your diet:

- Sodas
- Fried foods
- Sweet stuff—candy, cookies, cakes, etc.
- Processed food and meat
- Meat and dairy (okay in moderation)

You should try to curtail your visits to fast food restaurants and don't give your kids a treat by taking them there. What you are doing is conditioning them to see junk food as something it definitely is not. We will return to the subject of food, especially good food, in Chapter 19 on nutrition.

You are probably already doing some good things but if you are not doing enough you need to make sure that the pendulum is swinging firmly in the good direction. You will be amazed at how much you will enjoy and appreciate good health once you have it. You won't even know how bad you were feeling until you start feeling better! Most people don't realize that fatigue, digestive disorders, aches and pains, allergies and headaches are all early indicators of disease that can disable and kill.

According to Doctor Mark Hyman, one of my favorite health authors, conventional medicine helps when one is in the final stages of disease, but it is the wrong road for chronic illnesses because it does very little to treat the underlying causes. Diseases like diabetes and Alzheimer's start many years before they are conclusively diagnosed but we now know that good lifestyle choices can stop diabetes and at least slow down the onset of Alzheimer's.

The bottom line is that you really need to take a holistic approach to your health and implement the **Four Key Drivers** in your life. Let me remind you what they are:

1. **Exercise** is your "secret sauce" and must be a high priority for the rest of your life.

2. **Nutrition** is also very important and we will explore this further in Chapter 19.

3. **The X Factor** is your new lifestyle mission.

4. **Knowledge** about exercise, nutrition and health is the fourth key driver; your health is the focus of this chapter and the next. I briefly review the importance of sleep, deep breathing and the outdoors, as well as my favorite health books and authors, before we move on to Chapter 18—"Mind Your Brain".

The Importance of Sleep

Sleep is critical for good health and is probably as important as exercise and nutrition. You should aim to sleep between seven and nine hours a night, with an average of eight hours being ideal. When you cheat your body of the sleep it needs, your health will suffer and the risk of weight gain, diabetes, heart disease, strokes and premature aging increases. If you regularly sleep less than seven hours a night you are more likely to be overweight or obese. There is a strong negative relationship between food and sleep. The less sleep you get, the more you tend to eat; this helps to explain why there is such a compelling link between insomnia and diabetes.

When you are tired, you should go to sleep so that you don't set yourself up to make poor decisions. You should definitely not rely on energy drinks or medications to keep you awake longer. It is also important that you do not give up your sleep to fit in exercise; both are essential.

Here are a few ideas to help you get the ideal eight hours of sleep.

1. Try to control the time you go to bed; set your alarm to remind you when it is bedtime.

2. Try to be consistent about when you go to bed. For example, go to your bedroom at 9:00pm, turn the light out at 10:00pm, get up at 6:00am, eight hours later.

3. Make sure your bedroom is dark and quiet when you are sleeping. Try to eliminate any distracting lights or noises.

4. You can measure the quality of your sleep by dividing your total sleep time by your total time in bed. You should try to achieve 85% if possible.

Deep Breathing and the Outdoors

You should recognize by now that I am a big fan of exercising outdoors. I realize that the weather can be a limiting factor but in general, the more time you can spend outdoors, the better. You will nearly always feel good and you are much more likely to enjoy your exercise. The sun is a great source of vitamin D, though you do need to take care. The last thing you want to do is get skin cancer, so make sure you apply sunscreen as needed.

Exercise provides some great opportunities for deep breathing. When you increase the intensity of your exercise, you will automatically breathe more deeply as your breathing becomes heavier. The more oxygen you can get deep into your lungs to enrich your circulation, your heart and your brain, the better.

Deep breathing at any time is also a great way to calm yourself and energize your body. A good deep breathing technique is to sit comfortably, breathe in while you count slowly to five, hold your breath for another 5 and then breathe out for five. Repeat this for up to two minutes and see if you notice a difference.

My Favorite Health Books and Authors

Since I started my new mission to Get America Moving, I have read many books about health. It is clearly a very broad subject and well beyond the scope of *The eXercise Factor*. Consequently, I am pleased to share with you the books and authors that have made the greatest impression on me and I certainly recommend that you put them on your reading list.

1. *Younger Next Year—A guide to living like you're fifty until you're eighty and beyond.* By Chris Crowley and Henry S. Lodge, M.D. *Younger Next Year* shows you how to turn back your biological clock and become functionally younger every year for years to come and continue to live with vitality and grace into your eighties and beyond. It shows you how to avoid seventy percent of the decay and fifty percent of the injuries and illnesses associated with getting older.

2. *Use Your Brain To Change Your Age—Secrets to look, feel and think younger every day.* By Daniel G. Amen, M.D. A healthy brain is the key to staying vibrant and alive for a long time and in this New York Times bestseller, Dr. Amen shares ten simple steps to boost your brain to help you live longer, look younger and dramatically decrease your risk for Alzheimer's disease.

3. *The Blood Sugar Solution—The Ultra healthy program for losing weight, preventing disease and feeling great now!* By Mark Hyman, M.D. In *The Blood Sugar Solution*, Dr. Hyman presents his scientifically based program for rebalancing insulin and blood sugar levels. He identifies seven factors in achieving wellness and outlines his six-week action plan that gives you the tools you need to personalize your approach to healing.

4. *Eat to Live—The amazing nutrient-rich program for fast and sustained weight loss.* By Joel Fuhrman, M.D. *Eat to Live* offers a highly effective, scientifically proven way to lose weight quickly. The key to Dr. Furman's revolutionary six-week plan is a simple equation: health = nutrients/calories. When the ratio of nutrients to calories in the food you eat is high, you lose weight. The more nutrient dense food you eat, the less you crave fats, sweets and high calorie foods. Dr. Furman has just released a new book with a great title—*The End of Dieting!*

5. *The Great Cholesterol Myth—Why lowering your cholesterol won't prevent heart disease and the statin-free plan that will.* By Jonny Bowden, PH.D., C.N.S. and Stephen Sinatra, M.D., F.A.C.C. According to the authors, cholesterol and saturated fats don't cause heart disease; traditional heart disease protocols have gotten it all wrong. Science is showing that cholesterol and saturated fats are not a direct path to heart disease and that the standard prescription of low-fat diets and statin drugs are contributing to a health crisis of monumental proportions.

6. *Food Is Better Medicine Than Drugs—Your prescription for drug-free health.* By Patrick Holford and Jerome Burne. The authors expose the truth about prescription drugs and why we swallow what the drug industry tells us. They explain why the right combination of foods,

supplements and simple lifestyle changes offer long-term, drug-free solutions with immediate benefits to your health.

Good health does not come from doctors. They don't know everything and you don't have to do everything they tell you but I strongly recommend that you collaborate with a good primary care doctor on a regular basis.

Life is precious but it is also finite. Your time and your health are your most valuable assets but often a person doesn't fully recognize and appreciate this until they are nearly gone. You cannot simply buy extra quality time when you are sick but you can significantly extend your time by preventing disease in the first place.

Good health gives you the strength and energy to do what you want to do and it is never too late to get started. Dr. Daniel Amen was once asked, "I am sixty-five years old; is it too late to start?" He replied, "Only if you plan to live to sixty-six. If you want to live until you are ninety or beyond, now would be a good time to start."

And so I say to you—Now is a good time to start!

✗ Your "To Do" List

1. Develop a short list of the foods that you are going to avoid or at least minimize from your diet.

2. Develop another list of the actions you are going to take, including sleep, breathing and exercise outdoors, to make sure the pendulum is swinging firmly in the right direction.

3. Make sure that you take a holistic approach to your health and implement the four key drivers in your life.

4. Read more and increase your knowledge about health. Consider the list of my favorite books and authors.

"If someone is going down the wrong road,
he doesn't need motivation to speed him up.
What he needs is education to turn him around."
—Jim Rohn

CHAPTER 18

MIND YOUR BRAIN

I don't know about you, but until recently I never really thought about my brain. To be honest, it was a bit of a mystery to me and I think I just took it for granted. I am lucky that I don't suffer from headaches, except the increasingly rare, self-inflicted hangover. So think about this for a moment: I never use the thing I think with to think about the thing I think with. That's a useful tongue twister, which is also a good exercise for my thing!

All right, enough about my thing. Let's start talking about your thing, I mean, your brain. Have you ever thought about your brain? I mean, have you ever really thought about how it operates up there inside your skull, behind your eyes? If you think about it, as I have recently, you will realize that your brain is an organ which is actively involved in everything you do and every decision you make. I think we have a tendency to take our brains for granted and assume that they will just keep running as smoothly as a well-oiled machine—a bit like our hearts!

When was the last time you heard someone talk about their brain the way they might talk about other organs? Men talk about their prostates and women talk about their breasts and we all talk about our hearts. Don't get me wrong, it is important that we talk about these things. My question, though, is why don't we talk about our brains in the same way?

Your brain is a key organ and you need to look after it. I believe that your brain deserves the same attention as your heart, assuming you look after your heart. If not, they both require your immediate attention. Think about it this way. You will probably survive so long as your heart continues to operate. However, fortunately or unfortunately depending on your point of view, increasing numbers of people are surviving without a fully functional brain. Honestly, though, what is the point if your heart is working but your brain isn't? Not a lot to look forward to there, but here is some good news. Most of the things you need to do to look after your heart will benefit your brain as well. So that gives you double the motivation; you need to take actions which will benefit both your heart and your brain.

As part of my ongoing research, I have learned a lot about the brain. I recently had the privilege of attending a "brain" presentation by Dr. Daniel Amen, one of the world's leading authorities on the subject. Doctor Amen opened my eyes (or should I say my brain!) and has been a catalyst in developing my understanding of the subject. One of my objectives in this book is to share with you what I have learned and what I believe you need to know, too. However, I also encourage you to develop your own knowledge and understanding of the brain.

Some Important Facts

- Your brain is the most complex organ in your body, with around one hundred billion neurons, that's 100,000,000,000 give or take! That is more connections than there are stars in the universe! On average, we lose some eighty-five thousand neurons every day.
- Your brain represents about 2% of your body weight yet uses on average around 30% of your calories and 20% of your oxygen and blood flow. It is composed of around 75% water.
- Mild Cognitive Impairment (MCI) causes a slight but noticeable and measurable decline in cognitive abilities, including memory and thinking

skills. While personality remains intact, frequent memory lapses occur. A person with MCI is at an increased risk of developing Alzheimer's or another form of dementia.

- "Dementia" is an umbrella term used to describe a loss of cognitive function. It is often caused by a stroke or some other trauma to the brain. Alzheimer's is the most common form of dementia.

Alzheimer's Disease

According to the Alzheimer's Association, Alzheimer's disease is now an epidemic in the US. More than five million Americans have the disease today but the statistics are even more alarming. Someone develops Alzheimer's every 68 seconds and the total number of sufferers is projected to triple by 2050.

Alzheimer's will cost the USA some $200 billion in 2014 and this is projected to increase to $1.2 trillion by 2050. The average annual per capita cost of treating Alzheimer's is currently around $45,000 and when residential care is added it increases to $70,000. By any standard this is very significant and is a national financial disaster in waiting. Even worse, however, are the incalculable personal costs to families affected by this disease.

Alzheimer's is a progressive disease and is eventually fatal. It is the only one of the top ten causes of death in the USA that cannot be cured. What is really scary is that Alzheimer's disease actually starts some thirty years before the first symptoms show, so you must get on a prevention program *now*. According to Doctor Amen, this is an illness you do not want to get!

The question of whether Alzheimer's can be prevented continues to intrigue researchers and fuel ongoing investigations. While there are no clear-cut answers so far, many experts believe that you can prevent Alzheimer's by stopping or preventing all diseases associated with it, including heart disease, cancer, diabetes, depression and sleep apnea. In particular, controlling cardiovascular risk factors may be the most cost-effective and helpful approach to protecting brain health. In other words, if you have a healthy heart, there is a strong chance you will have a healthy brain and can thus avoid dementia, including Alzheimer's. The best news of all is that you can choose to take actions which will help you avoid becoming a statistic in this chilling epidemic.

Motivation for a Healthy Brain

What are the most important things in life? As we learned earlier, when asked this question, most people will answer either their family or their health and that is hardly a surprise. What is surprising, however, is how few of these people make the real live connection between their family and their health and put in place a set of objectives and plans designed to ensure there is congruence between them.

I would like to live a long and happy life and I want to do that with my wife, my kids, my family, and my friends. I certainly don't want to lose my connection with or be a burden to the people I love, at any time in the future. While I cannot guarantee this outcome, there is an awful lot I can do to reduce the risks and improve my chances.

High Performance Brain

Clearly it is a huge mistake to ignore your brain because the quality of your decisions is directly linked to its health. If you have a healthy brain you are likely to be happier, healthier, more successful and make better decisions. On the other hand, if you have an unhealthy brain you are likely to be sadder, sicker, less successful and make poor decisions.

If you could develop a high performance brain plan to boost your brain and slow or even reverse the aging process, would you? I hope so, as taking these actions will not only help your brain but improve everything else in your life as well. When your brain works properly, so do you. Conversely, when it has trouble you do, too.

According to Doctor Amen your goal should be to develop "brain envy". In other words, think about your brain the same way many people think about their bodies with envy—men desiring a slim, muscular body with a six-pack or women craving a body that could be a top model.

While your brain typically becomes less active as you age over time, you have the choice to have either a healthy or an unhealthy brain. We know that current average life expectancy at age sixty-five is around eighty-two for men and eighty-five for women. However, in my view this could be and should be as much as fifteen years higher. Your new lifestyle mission requires both a great body and a great brain! You will need the energy and stamina required to sustain your mental capabilities. To be mentally slow at any age is not normal.

Reduce the Risks—What You Need To Avoid

Our behavior either accelerates brain aging or slows it down. It does one or the other so you should try to avoid things that might hurt your brain and in particular, things that will speed up the aging process. The more bad decisions you make now, the more likely you are to reduce the quality of your "golden" years. The first obstacle you need to overcome is the danger of not understanding your brain's vulnerability and the effect brain health has on the rest of your life. The following are major risks for the brain and you should try to avoid these at all costs:

- **Heart Disease:** All the problems associated with heart and blood circulation diseases increase the risks for our brain as well.
- **Obesity:** Overweight and obesity cause similar problems for the brain as they do for the heart. You want to avoid what Doctor Amen calls the "Dinosaur Syndrome"; a big body and a small brain. This is based on research done by Dr. Cyrus Raji from the University of Pittsburg which demonstrates that as our weight (especially our waist size) increases, the actual physical size of our brain decreases and brain function is impaired. Fat deposits in the body also store toxic materials which hinder the brain.
- **Pre-Diabetes:** Some people think pre-diabetes is not a problem until it becomes full-blown diabetes; it is just a warning sign. Nothing could be further from the truth! It is an early stage of the disease which carries the same risks as diabetes. Pre-diabetes can kill you too, through heart disease, stroke and even cancer. It can also cause pre-dementia or mild cognitive impairment—think of it as early Alzheimer's.
- **Diabetes:** Recent studies have shown that diabetics have four times the risk of developing Alzheimer's and patients with metabolic syndrome (pre-diabetes) have a dramatically increased risk of pre-dementia or mild cognitive impairment (MCI). You don't even have to have diabetes to have brain damage and memory loss from high insulin levels and insulin resistance. Alzheimer's disease is increasingly being referred to as type 3 diabetes.
- **Sleep Apnea:** This can be a serious problem, especially if linked to one or more of the above risks.

- **High Blood Pressure**: This causes progressive damage to the brain's structure and function, increasing the risk of stroke and dementia, including Alzheimer's disease.
- **Stress**: Chronic stress and depression cause all sorts of problems for the brain, from mild cognitive impairment to an increased risk for Alzheimer's disease.
- **Bad Food**: A poor diet, especially if it includes a lot of junk food, is a major problem as it can lead to cancer, heart disease, diabetes, obesity, depression, dementia, etc.
- **Sugar:** This is such a major problem for the whole body that it deserves separate mention from bad food. Sugar is addictive, causes inflammation and leads to a whole host of problems for the brain.
- **Bad Fats:** This includes trans fats and too much saturated fat; together they cause major problems for the body and the brain.
- **Caffeine**: This restricts blood flow and dehydrates you; remember the brain is around 75% water. Coffee or black tea in moderation is fine but remember—caffeine is addictive which can lead to drinking too much of it. Also, according to Doctor Amen, anything that results in withdrawal symptoms is not your friend.
- **Smoking**: This starves the brain of oxygen and prematurely ages the brain in the same way as it ages your skin.
- **Alcohol:** Red wine is fine for your heart, in small doses. However, according to Doctor Amen, all forms of alcohol are bad for your brain. I love red wine, so I'll be honest and say that this is a big challenge for me!
- **Metals:** Too much exposure to metals such as iron, copper or aluminum, as well as other toxic substances lead to oxidation, and the resulting free radicals cause problems for the brain.
- **Medicine:** Prescription medications, such as statins and sleeping pills, as well as many over-the-counter medications can have adverse effects on your brain and especially your memory. Unfortunately, no one is really tracking this so always start with other healthy options, including good food, as your solution before you take medicine. Even then, keep your medication to a minimum.

It is important to react to problems by going toward health rather than running away from it. If you fall into one or more of the above categories, you are not doing your brain any favors and you need to take positive action right away.

Improve Your Chances—What You Need To Do

I referred to this in the last section but it is worth repeating—you must start by taking your brain seriously and make sure you know about the health of your brain. I have just covered the things you need to avoid; here now are several positive actions you can take to help your brain:

- **Exercise:** Surprise! Surprise! Physical activity is as important for your brain as it is for your heart. Aerobic exercise directly benefits the brain by increasing blood and oxygen flow, bringing nutrients and taking waste away. Building up your muscle strength is also crucial to reducing the risk of Alzheimer's. However, the strongest evidence derives from exercise's proven benefits to the cardiovascular system, which we now know also benefits the brain.

- **Cognitive Exercise:** This is equally important in reducing and possibly delaying age-related shrinkage of your brain. Keep your brain active by continuous learning, reading and testing or training of your memory.

- **Good Food:** Your brain uses 30% of all the calories you consume but it is not a simple "calories in versus calories out" equation. It should be *high quality* calories in, including foods that are high in fiber, have lower glycemic indexes and/or contain healthy fats, versus *high quality* energy out. However, just like exercise, your diet may have its greatest impact on brain health through its effect on heart health.

- **Good Fat:** While you want to avoid bad fats, a low-fat diet is also unhealthy for you. Some 50% of the solid weight of your brain, after taking water out, is made up of fat so make sure you consume good, healthy fats from natural foods such as salmon, avocados, walnuts, etc.

- **Water:** Your brain is made up of around 75% water, so it should be pretty obvious that hydration is just as important, if not more important, for the brain than any other part of the body.

- **Sleep:** Your body needs to rest and sleep and so does your brain. You need to get at least seven hours and preferably an average of eight hours of sleep a night so that your brain has enough time to complete some of its "backing up" tasks, including memory—just like your computer. Try to limit your intake of both caffeine and alcohol as they can adversely affect the quality of your sleep. Don't make important decisions when you are tired.

- **Stress Management:** As we know that stress causes all kinds of problems for the brain, we need to take affirmative action to manage the stress in our lives. Doctor Amen refers to ANT (automatic negative thoughts) killing. You need to manage and control these sad, mad and nervous thoughts; the answer to ANTS, according to Doctor Amen, is to write them down and talk back to yourself!

- **Supplements:** You should get as many as possible of the vitamins and minerals your body needs from natural foods rather than vitamin pills. Vitamin E (found in spinach, sweet potatoes, nuts and seeds) is particularly important because it may significantly reduce the risk of Alzheimer's. B Vitamins (specifically B6, Folic Acid and B12), which you get from a diverse range of whole foods, may reduce brain atrophy as well as preserve and even help you improve your memory.

- **Antioxidants:** These deserve special mention as they can significantly improve your overall brain health. They help fight oxidation, a normal chemical process that takes place in the body and the brain every day. When there are disruptions in the natural oxidation process, highly unstable and potentially damaging molecules called free radicals are created. Oxygen triggers the formation of these destructive chemicals, and, if left uncontrolled, they can cause damage to cells in the brain. It's much like the chemical reaction that creates rust on a bicycle or turns the surface of a cut apple brown. Antioxidants and free radicals can be explained by visualizing your circulation as a highway. Sometimes there are cracks and potholes in the road. Free radicals are like the cracks in the road and the antioxidants are the stuff used to fill the holes and make the road normal again. You can get all the antioxidants you need from a diet containing plenty of fruits, vegetables, whole grains and nuts.

By taking the above actions you can significantly improve the functioning of your brain and reverse the aging process. You need to control both your body and your brain for the rest of your life; they are inextricably linked.

✗ Your "To Do" List

I have set out five key actions you should implement immediately to develop a proactive brain culture in your life below.

1. Develop your knowledge and education
    a. Honor, respect and care for your brain as much as you do your heart
    b. Use images of family to reinforce your decision to be brain-healthy
2. Make exercise an important part of your life
    a. Aerobic exercise
    b. Muscle strengthening
    c. Increase intensity
3. Develop brain-healthy nutrition as your way of life.
    a. Never buy bad food that will hurt others, especially kids
    b. Be a friend—not an accomplice
4. Focus on your brain as a key component of your new lifestyle mission
    a. Inspire others, especially your family, to join in
    b. Set an example for your kids

Make sure you get eight hours of sleep and pay serious attention to your hydration. See the section called "Drink Plenty of Water" in the next chapter on Nutrition.

Footnote: You need to acquire as much knowledge as you can about the physical health of your brain, but how will you learn unless you look? According to Doctor Amen, brain scans will be as common as colonoscopies by 2020. You will learn a lot about your brain at Brain Fit Life, including details about brain health assessments based on scores and exercises that enhance your brain. Go to **www.MyBrainFitLife.com**.

"Physical fitness is not only one of the most important keys to a healthy body; it is the basis of dynamic and creative intellectual activity."
—John F. Kennedy

CHAPTER 19

NUTRITION—YOUR FOURTH KEY DRIVER

lthough nutrition is not my area of expertise, I spend considerable time reading about, studying and researching this area because I need to know more. With the guidance and help of my lovely wife Maureen, who has recently completed a health coach training program with the Institute for Integrative Nutrition, this research has really opened my eyes into the many issues we face on the food and nutrition front. I really believe we have major problems with the Inactivity Epidemic, but things are at least as bad, if not worse, in the area of food and nutrition.

Changes in My Lifetime

Like so many other things, how we eat has changed dramatically in my lifetime. When I was growing up back in the sixties and seventies, our eating and drinking habits were vastly different. First of all, the variety of food available was much smaller and thus we had a more basic diet than we do now. There were also no fast food restaurants, at least not in Ireland, and we seldom, if ever, ate in what we perceived as "fancy" restaurants.

Breakfast was always an important meal of the day and usually included half an orange (not orange juice), porridge or oatmeal, whole-grain brown bread and tea. Coffee only became popular in Ireland in the eighties.

Lunch was called dinner because it was the main meal of the day and simple economics dictated that a small portion (four or five ounces) of lean meat or fish was accompanied by plenty of potatoes and vegetables. This was usually followed by dessert, which was often homemade; we called it "sweet" for obvious reasons.

The third meal of the day was called tea, which I assume got its name from the drink. Yes, we did drink hot tea, usually with milk added; sugar was an optional extra which I am pleased to say I stopped using at an early age. This was a relatively small meal around 6:00pm; maybe toasted cheese or scrambled eggs with some hot scones, butter and strawberry or raspberry jam. We usually had a fourth meal as well, called supper, about an hour before bed. Depending on the time of year, this was usually a glass of cold milk or a cup of cocoa (hot chocolate) with a couple of wholegrain cookies.

What is very interesting to me now as I reflect back on that time is how much better things were. Breakfast was always very important, dinner was eaten in the middle of the day, portions were much smaller and we ate many more whole foods, fruits and vegetables than we do now.

My dad would regularly go to Dublin's wholesale market and buy large boxes of fruits and vegetables. We had a vegetable garden, as well as some apple and pear trees, in our backyard. We were not unusual; many people did the same. Milk was delivered every day to our door in glass bottles by the "milkman", bread was delivered a few times a week by the "breadman" and eggs were delivered by a man called Joe. We drank cold milk with our meals (though I never really liked it) and plenty of tap water whenever we were thirsty. There was no bottled water! Did we feel deprived? Never!

Christmas Day

Another personal memory, which vividly illustrates the huge changes between then and now, took place each Christmas Day. For kids, this was the number one celebration of the year. As a special treat for Christmas dinner, my parents would buy a large bottle of Cidona, a fizzy apple drink which was shared between four children. We looked forward to this all year but when that bottle of soda was gone, it was gone for another year.

Much of this was dictated by simple economics, for when it came to diet and nutrition my parents were no smarter than parents today, but intuitively they knew what was good and what was bad for us. Remember, they did not know what we know now about our food and nutrition. On the other hand, they also were not bombarded with confusing and conflicting information every day.

America's Food Culture

I am not sure if it was always this way, but when it comes to food portions in America, size definitely matters. Everywhere you go portions are "super-sized" and it appears that supply and demand are in close harmony with each other; that is, consumers demand the portion sizes provided by restaurants.

Television is saturated with popular programs such as *Man Versus Food*, *United States of Bacon* and *America's Manliest Restaurants*, all of which glorify eating huge portions of food. These television shows reinforce the notion that you are not a man unless you can devour huge portions of food, especially meat.

There is no question that meat is usually the main attraction. Steak portions are now so big that it is very difficult to find a restaurant which serves a small steak under six ounces, which would be considered a healthy portion. Eight ounces is nearly always the smallest size and twelve, sixteen and twenty-four-ounce steaks are common, with no upper limit. Consumers are looking for bigger steaks and there are restaurants all over America with steak-eating challenges of gigantic proportions.

Popular Restaurants

Whereas eating out was the exception rather than the rule when I was growing up, it is probably fair to say that for most Americans it is now part of everyday life. Most popular restaurants, especially those in the low-to-moderate price range, which cater to the vast majority of consumers, truly believe more is better.

All-you-can-eat buffets are now very popular. In most other restaurants, the appetizers are big enough to be entrées and most entrées are big enough to be shared, or at least to be cut in half, with half brought home in a doggy bag for tomorrow's dinner (or perhaps, in some cases, the dog). My wife Maureen regularly orders an appetizer with a vegetable side instead of an entrée and occasionally we share an entrée.

While a large meat portion is the star attraction on the vast majority of restaurant menus, next in line is the carbohydrates. These are usually French fries, baked potatoes or pasta, with an unlimited supply of bread (usually white) at the start. In some restaurants, meat by itself is the entrée, with carbs and vegetables cast in the role of optional extras. There is often not a vegetable in sight and when there is, it usually plays a supporting role in the "sides" category. With portions already way too big, there is little incentive to order what is probably considered by many as nothing more than an unnecessary additional expenditure, even though these vegetables are essential for vitamins and minerals.

When you order a soda your server will probably keep filling your glass unless you tell them otherwise. They understandably perceive this as an easy way to provide you with great service and enhance their tip, so you can't blame the server. Keep a close eye on this the next time you order a soda in a restaurant, or you, or perhaps even worse, your kids, could consume an additional one thousand calories without really thinking about it!

While diet sodas do eliminate the calories, though not the caffeine, they are not a good solution because the calories are replaced with artificial sweeteners which fulfill your craving for something sweet. The problem is that these fake sugars tease and confuse your body so it doesn't release the necessary hormones that regulate your blood sugar. This is one of the reasons why so many diet soda drinkers continue to have weight problems. Don't let all that ice trick you either; the glass is also much bigger than it used to be.

Standard American Diet is Killing Our Kids

This is a provocative statement which I believe is true, but let me clarify. I am sure that most Americans do not intentionally make themselves sick through eating too much of the wrong food. I am also absolutely certain that the vast majority of American parents are not intentionally condemning their kids to a life of obesity, diabetes and premature death.

Recently, I was standing in line for breakfast at one of my favorite coffee shops when I noticed a little boy—well, a pretty big boy actually. He was six, maybe seven years old, definitely overweight and probably obese. He had a plate of pancakes, nicely cut up into small, bite-sized pieces and he had a fork in his hand. His dad was standing over him, pouring maple syrup onto his pancakes and they both had big smiles on their faces. They were having a great time. I had no doubt whatsoever that the dad truly loved his son and would never intentionally do him any harm!

Of course, my experience is not a unique one. Everywhere you go, whether in restaurants, hotels, or even at home, kids eat pancakes or waffles for breakfast. Very few eat the healthier alternatives of fruit and oatmeal anymore. When I was a kid, we had pancakes once a year, on what we called "Pancake" or "Shrove Tuesday", the day before Lent. These pancakes were similar to thin French crêpes and were served with a small sprinkle of sugar and lemon juice. A bit like the Cidona I mentioned earlier, this was an annual treat which I always looked forward to.

Over the years, my kids have been involved in many sports, including cross-country, track and field, swimming, soccer, field hockey and lacrosse. By any definition, these are all healthy pursuits. Unfortunately, however, the standard food and drink for the kids at all meets and tournaments is pizza, cookies, brownies, doughnuts and sodas, which include "sports" drinks and are also full of sugar. We can hardly blame the kids, if their parents and coaches consistently provide junk food and perpetuate the standard American diet.

Food Labeling And Serving Sizes

You need to be a scientist to read food labels today. There is no doubt in my mind that this is done purposely to confuse you; the aim of all companies is to maximize their profit and this is certainly more difficult to do if consumers eat less of their product! Beware of added sugar. It amazes me when I look at the ingredient lists of common foods, even things like spaghetti sauce, that sugar is added. If you were to make the spaghetti sauce yourself you would never think of adding sugar; who puts sugar on their entree? Increasingly, processed foods have added sugar, fat and salt.

When you look at say, a typical bag of chips, the serving size on the label is invariably small and there are many servings in the bag. So you have to look at the fine print to figure out how much you should consume and you will probably need a calculator to work out the calories. Given the fact that most of us do not have the time or inclination to do all that, our perception of serving sizes has, let's say evolved, over the years.

With bigger and bigger portions in restaurants, our understanding of what a serving size should be is totally distorted. Many meals are now served "family style", which means the portions are meant for sharing—not just for one person. Let's see how your portion sizes measure up; the following chart provides recommended portion sizes for various food groups.

HANDY GUIDELINE FOR PORTION CONROL

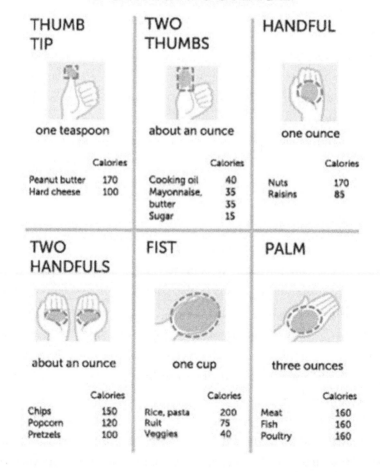

THUMB TIP

one teaspoon

	Calories
Peanut butter	170
Hard cheese	100

TWO THUMBS

about an ounce

	Calories
Cooking oil	40
Mayonnaise,	35
butter	35
Sugar	15

HANDFUL

one ounce

	Calories
Nuts	170
Raisins	85

TWO HANDFULS

about an ounce

	Calories
Chips	150
Popcorn	120
Pretzels	100

FIST

one cup

	Calories
Rice, pasta	200
Fruit	75
Veggies	40

PALM

three ounces

	Calories
Meat	160
Fish	160
Poultry	160

Nutrition versus Calories

Most weight loss diets are based on calories or points. While it is important to track the numbers, what if you looked at the nutritional value the food has to offer? Many people, especially men, are more concerned with what they put into their car than they are about what they put into their bodies. Assuming you want to live a high quality life for a long time, I'm sure you will agree that it makes sense to give more thought to what you put into your body and how you nourish it.

Let's use the chart above to compare a typical entree based on calorie count and nutritional value. An entree of one thousand Calories is made up as follows:

- 9 oz. steak with sauce—560 Calories
- Portion of baked potato—400 Calories
- Portion of vegetables—40 Calories

Now let's make a few changes so our focus is on the nutritional value of the meal as follows:

- 6 oz. steak with sauce—375 Calories
- One small portion of potatoes—200 Calories
- Double portion of vegetables—80 Calories

These changes ensure that while you still get sufficient protein, fat and carbohydrates you now get an increased percentage of vitamins, minerals and fiber from the extra vegetables. By focusing on nutrition, you can reduce the size of the steak and potatoes, double your vegetables and reduce the total calories from 1000 to 655. This is very significant if you want to lose weight and improve your health. You don't have to worry about feeling hungry, as the vegetables will fill you up. Even if you added a third portion of vegetables, you would still significantly reduce your total calories.

Consider the nutritional value of a one hundred calorie bar of chocolate compared to an apple. Not really a fair comparison is it, as most of us would probably prefer the bar of chocolate. It's not fair in another way either, as it is hard to find a one hundred calorie bar of chocolate and thus you have to discipline yourself to share it or save some for later!

The ingredients of chocolate bars usually include cocoa solids, cocoa butter, sugar, milk and, depending on the brand, other additives and flavorings. In contrast, an apple is a whole food in its original form, has around one hundred sixteen calories and a host of vitamins, minerals, natural sugar and fiber. The apple gives more of a nutritional "punch" to your body than the chocolate bar. So, knowing this, would you choose the apple or the chocolate? Maybe you would still sometimes choose the chocolate, but at least you are making an informed decision when you focus on the nutritional value of your food. Stopping to think about what you eat and what the food does for you will greatly affect the size of your waist and your wallet!

So what do you do now?

Fad diets come and go. Diets that restrict food intake based on calories or points are very difficult to sustain in the long-term. You must be able to continue your healthy new eating habits without a relapse. The biggest drawback to the majority of diets is that once it ends, the weight nearly always comes back. Your metabolism responds negatively to restrictive dieting and makes weight maintenance over time even more difficult than before. A much more effective approach is to focus on good, balanced nutrition which you can sustain for the rest of your life.

What is good, balanced nutrition?

Think whole foods. You can recognize whole foods very easily because they are always in their original form; they have not been processed or changed to look like something else. Consider your local supermarket, where you will find most whole foods, such as fruit, vegetables, meat, fish, eggs and dairy, around the perimeter of the store, although there are some, such as nuts and beans, which are usually located in the center aisles. Try to increase the amount of these fresh, whole foods and reduce the amount of the processed junk in your cart and you will be well on your way to having a more balanced and nutritious diet.

Breakfast is arguably the most important meal of the day, yet many people either skip it altogether or go for the fast food option. I like to keep it simple with some fruit, oatmeal or my favorite homemade wholegrain, Irish brown bread with some scrambled eggs for protein.

If you are used to eating out at lunchtime, you should consider packing a homemade lunch, at least a few days a week. Research studies show that people who eat in restaurants consume many more calories than those who prepare their own food. Chunky vegetable soup, a small sandwich with lean meat, using mustard instead of mayo for your condiment, and some fruit to finish would be a good balanced meal. When you have lunch in a restaurant, remember that sandwiches today are much bigger than they used to be, so ask for less meat and more salad or vegetables in your sandwich and you will get a better nutritional punch.

Drink Plenty of Water

You should drink plenty of water throughout the day because it is very good for you on numerous fronts. Dehydration is always your enemy, not just when it is hot outside but also during colder months when you don't feel as thirsty. Dehydration is not good for your heart, your circulation, your bones and especially your brain. You are also much more likely to reach for a soda to quench your thirst. You can easily tell when you are dehydrated by the color of your urine. The clearer it is, the more hydrated you are; the darker it is, the more dehydrated you are.

Because water is so important, I have set out seven simple actions which you can take to stay hydrated on a daily basis. As an added bonus, these actions will also help you lose or control your weight!

1. Drink plenty of water throughout the day. Tap or bottled water is good, filtered water is better and distilled water is best, because unwanted chemicals are eliminated.
2. Make sure your water is cold; your body will burn more calories warming up the cold water to its normal temperature.
3. Add a hint of flavor if you need to make your water taste better. A small wedge of lemon or lime is my favorite.
4. Drink a large glass of water before every meal and this will both aid digestion and stop you from overeating.

5. Eat plenty of water-rich fruit and vegetables.
6. Eat plenty of vegetable soup and drink smoothies made from real fruit.
7. Always drink water before, during and after exercise.

If you need to work on this, you should set up reminders that work for you. I would use simple post-it notes but you can certainly use one of the many more "technologically advanced" options available as well.

One last reason for drinking plenty of water and staying hydrated is that you will need to pee more often. By itself this is a good thing, as this is how your body eliminates waste. However, it also gives you the opportunity to take a five- or ten-minute break from work or whatever you are doing. The break will do you good and you can do some baseline exercise on your way to and from the bathroom.

Turbo Charge Your Metabolism

You can turbo charge your metabolism through a combination of effective exercise and good, balanced nutrition. If you are overweight, you probably need to reduce your calorie intake even if you increase your exercise. But you should aim to do this gradually and, as shown in the illustration above, you can significantly reduce your calories just by focusing on wholesome, sensible nutrition. Combined with your increased exercise, this will literally turbo charge your metabolism and will help you burn calories even faster.

Please make sure that your calorie reduction does not interfere with the effectiveness of your exercise. Yes, you heard that correctly. As you increase your exercise, your need for excellent quality nutrition increases, so the last thing you should do is reduce your food to the point where you have no energy left to do the additional exercise.

Refer to the graph in Chapter 3 which shows the relationship between exercise and calories. Ultimately, your objective is to find the right balance between your exercise and nutritional needs so that you can achieve your new long-term lifestyle mission.

Nutrition Influences Your Decisions

You can improve your ability to make good decisions by increasing your knowledge and creating the right environment for good decision-making. The top of the list here is wholesome nutrition, so your body can provide your brain with the right fuel at the right time.

Your body uses glucose when important decisions are required, so it is very important to make sure that both your body and brain are properly fueled before these decisions are made. As you know, you should go for whole foods like vegetables, nuts and fruits. Foods that are loaded with sugar, such as sodas and candy, may be the fastest way to get energy but they produce sugar peaks and troughs, leaving you short on glucose and on self-control.

You can eat your way to increased self-control and better decision-making. This is why you should always eat a good breakfast—especially on days when you're likely to be physically or mentally stressed. If you have an important meeting, interview or exam, don't take it on without properly fueling your body and brain first.

I believe this also reinforces my belief that dieting is generally not a good idea. If you significantly restrict your calorie intake, which most diets do, then by definition you are making it much more difficult to make good decisions. This may help to explain why so many diets fail—folks lack the necessary fuel needed to produce the willpower required to make the decisions needed to keep the diet going.

This also reinforces my view that the combination of vigorous exercise and restrictive dieting does not work well together. Not only are you short on fuel for the exercise but you are also low on the willpower required to follow through with good decisions.

✗ Your "To Do" List

As everyone needs to control their weight, your "to do" list focuses on the most important actions you can take to achieve this.

1. Turbo charge your metabolism through a combination of effective exercise and good, balanced nutrition.

2. Focus on food which you can enjoy for the rest of your life. Increase the amount of fresh, whole foods you eat and reduce the quantity of processed junk.

3. If you are trying to lose weight, do not let calorie reduction interfere with your capacity to exercise. It took time for your weight to increase, so be patient as it decreases.

4. Drink plenty of water throughout the day and in doing so, reduce the temptation to drink sodas, including diet sodas.

5. When it comes to eating, try to start the day big and end small. You should never skip breakfast, as this will only sabotage your weight loss efforts.

6. Make sure you have a healthy, nutritionally-balanced lunch. If you do, you will be less likely to snack during the day or eat a huge dinner in the evening.

7. When it is time for dinner, you will be ready to follow the illustration in this chapter—small portions of protein and carbs with plenty of vegetables.

"Don't start a diet that has an expiration date,
focus on a lifestyle that will last forever."
—Unknown

CHAPTER 20

HOW TO START EXERCISE IN 5 EASY STEPS

I f you have gotten this far in the book, then I am confident that I have persuaded you that exercise is a critical part of the solution to our health problems, not only in the USA, but all across the world. The evidence is overwhelming that exercise will help you increase your life expectancy and with it, the quality of your life as well. So whether you are doing too little exercise or no exercise at all, there is no better time than the present and that means <u>today</u>, or tomorrow if you are reading this late at night, to get started!

I feel so strongly about this subject that I created my very own health and fitness motto which allows me to reinforce this message again and again. Here it is:

"You don't need to be fit and healthy to start but you do need to START to be fit and healthy!"

217

The word **START** is self-explanatory, but in this chapter I use it as an easy-to-remember acronym which shows you "How to Start Exercise in 5 Easy Steps". I have addressed much of this already earlier in the book but I wanted to pull it all together into five easy steps.

I have used this acronym about starting to exercise on many occasions and if you would like to see one of my television interviews you can find these on my YouTube Channel: **www.Youtube.com/user/GetAmericaMoving1/videos**.

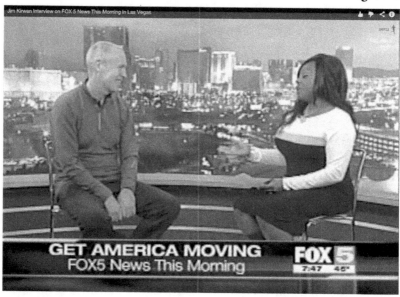

"S" is for Show Up

This sounds obvious, doesn't it? Yet while I have discussed this before, it is such a simple principle that I repeat it here in this chapter. In all my years involved with exercise, this is probably the *single biggest factor* in whether you will succeed or fail. Show up and you are halfway there; fail to show up and you will fail!

While "showing up" is always critical to success, it is especially true when you are starting. It is extraordinarily important to start off well. If you fail to achieve your short-term goals, as sure as night follows day, you will also fail to achieve your medium and longer-term goals. Get into the habit of showing up in the early days and you will have set yourself up for success.

I already mentioned the Walking and Running Club in Mount Pleasant that started in 2012. Remember how I pointed out that out of some five hundred folks who initially signed up as members, only fifty showed up with any regularity? Well, these fifty are making incredible strides forward with their health and fitness. The moral of the story is that you have to take action to achieve your project goals and if you just show up, amazing things can happen!

"T" is for Time

Again, it sounds very obvious but you have to allocate some of your precious and scarce time to your exercise if you want to succeed. The greatest obstacle to exercise is lack of time and the most common reason people give for not exercising is that they don't have enough time. So you really have to ask yourself where exactly exercise ranks in your list of priorities. If it is low, I think it helps to take a few minutes to figure out why you are where you are. Low priorities tend to be the ones that get discarded when the pressure comes on and "you don't have enough time". If you really want to start exercising and be assured of success you need to see it as a much higher priority in your life.

If you have a better understanding of the risks associated with *not* exercising and more importantly, the many benefits you will experience when you *do* exercise, you are more likely to promote exercise to the high priority level it deserves. Once it is higher on your priority list, it will be much easier to allocate the appropriate amount of time required for your exercise. Ideally, you need to get into the habit of exercising at certain times of the week. For example, I always run on Saturday and Sunday mornings. During the week, however, depending on the time of year, I exercise either early in the morning when it is hot or later in the afternoon when it is cold.

I also encourage you, especially at the start, to make appointments with yourself or your exercise partner and record these in your journal. You can schedule these a week or two in advance but it would be preferable to plan for the month ahead and roll this forward every week.

Exercise will help you to prioritize and manage your time and compel you to be more organized. There are twenty-four hours in every day and one hundred sixty-eight hours in every week. If you designate exercise as a high priority in your life then finding between three (the minimum) and seven (the optimum) hours each week to exercise shouldn't be that difficult.

"A" is for Accountable

You are accountable for your actions and you have to understand and accept the fact that ultimately the buck stops with you. This is crucial because if you do not embrace this reality, it is highly unlikely that you will achieve your goals.

It often helps to find someone else who will hold you accountable. It should be someone you trust and respect but also someone who is firm enough not to accept excuses from you if you start to waiver. This person could be your coach, personal trainer, exercise partner or family member. It is always much harder to break a commitment that you have made to someone else.

It also helps to record details of *what* you are going to do as well as *how* and *when* you are going to do it. We covered this project planning and goal setting extensively in Part 3. You should definitely write all of this down in your journal or diary and if you don't have one yet, you should get one as soon as possible to help you stay accountable. You should also get your accountability partner to sign off and confirm what you have agreed to in writing.

There is also a lot to be said for "public" goal setting, which really just means telling people what you are planning to do. As we have discussed before, by doing this you are much more likely to succeed, probably because of the fear of embarrassment you may feel if you do not deliver. In a sense, you feel more accountable for achieving your goals when you involve other people. Another great way to do this is to select your favorite charity and ask them if you can raise some money for them doing whatever you are planning to do and then tell the world—you are unlikely to fail!

"R" is for Results

It is really important to think carefully about the results that you want to achieve when you start exercising. What exactly do you want to accomplish? Do you want to get fit and improve your overall health? Do you want to lose weight, run a race, prepare for a bike trip, get ready for your ski vacation? Whatever it is, the more you can visualize the outcome the better; this allows you to reverse engineer your project plan and goals.

When you have a clear picture of the project result you desire, working backwards it is relatively easy to decide on your overall objectives. As the popular saying goes, if you fail to plan, prepare to fail. Preparation really is half the battle and every project you undertake requires a detailed plan in order to be successful. Your plan is really a road map of how you are going to get from point A, where you are now, to point B, where you want to be at some point in the future.

Setting goals is important as they give you clear direction. This well-defined path—where you are going and how you are going to get there—significantly increases your chances of a successful outcome. It always helps to break down your overall objective (your desired result) into smaller steps or milestones along the way, so you know that you are on track and heading in the right direction. Your goals need to be effective—by that I mean that they are set up in a way that maximizes the likelihood that you will achieve them. Refer to the section on how to set effective goals using the acronym **S.M.A.R.T.** in Chapter 14.

"T" is for Towel

It is vitally important that you never "throw in the towel". Unfortunately, many people do, maybe because they feel their exercise is too hard or they are not making any progress. It is important to understand and accept that exercise is hard work, particularly at the start. This is, of course, intensified if you are older or overweight, or if you have been inactive for some time. You should therefore see it as a challenge which will take time, but also a challenge at which you <u>will</u> succeed if you persevere and stick at it.

Let me give you another illustration with which I hope you will identify. Each year the *Biggest Loser* competition has a new set of participants who are very happy to be selected, even though they know they have a daunting task ahead. However, within a few weeks of starting, things begin to change rapidly. We see the participants getting sick, falling off machines, crying and generally behaving like babies. They are all stretched to their limits and close to throwing in the towel.

Now picture them at the end of the competition; they are totally transformed and even more highly motivated than they were at the start. They have worked their way through the competition and have succeeded. Everyone involved is very proud of themselves, and rightly so!

This can happen for you, too! Perhaps you won't have all the fanfare but you can definitely succeed just as others have done. You have to take on the challenge, accepting that it will be hard but being absolutely determined to persevere when times get tough. And always believe that you, too will achieve the outcome you are looking for.

Conclusion

Use the START acronym to help you get started with your exercise, whatever it is, today. Get into the habit of showing up and make exercise a high priority in your life. If you do this, finding time for it will not be a problem. Ultimately you are accountable but find someone else who will hold you to it and not accept excuses. Focus on the result you want to achieve and whatever you do, never throw in the towel. Keep working and persevere; you will be successful!

The 30-Day Exercise Challenge

A great way for you to start exercise is to complete the Get America Moving 30-Day Exercise Challenge. I created this FREE Challenge for this very reason and you can get immediate access to it at **www.GetAmericaMoving.com/challenge**. Make sure you watch the short video on my website homepage before you sign up.

When you sign up you will immediately receive an email with another short welcome video. This email and video outline three challenge options for you to choose from, based on <u>your current level of fitness</u> as set out in the table below.

Current Activity	Program 1*	Program 2	Program 3
Days per week	Inactive	2–3	3–4
Hours per week	Inactive	1–2	2–3
Aerobic Activity	Inactive	Walking	Walking
Speed (MPH)	Inactive	Less than 3	More than 3
Pace (Mins. Per Mile)	Inactive	20+	17+

* Inactive for 30 days or more

You simply select the program option that is right for you and when you do, you will receive the appropriate guidelines to help you get the most out of your 30-Day Exercise Challenge.

Get Ready For Some Major Changes

The Challenge is evergreen, which means you can start it at any time. However, I encourage you to get started right away and make this investment in your lifestyle, your life expectancy and your future quality of life. If you do this, you will have made a great decision and I am very confident that you will make remarkable progress on your journey with the 30-Day Exercise Challenge.

The Challenge is not difficult, but it definitely requires both effort and perseverance. Thirty days may seem like a major commitment—and it is!—but it is a necessary one which will enable you to get into the habit of exercising. Additionally, thirty days will also give you enough time to see significant improvements in your fitness level. It will be well worth the effort, because by the end of the thirty days, you will see that getting fit and healthy, while challenging, are absolutely realistic goals. You'll establish the habit of exercise in your life and your confidence will soar because you've set yourself up for continued success. You will want to continue the new lifestyle journey you have started and together we will "Get America Moving"!

✗ Your "To Do" List

1. Use the S.T.A.R.T. acronym to help you start exercising today.
2. Make exercise a high priority in your life and get into the habit of showing up.
3. Focus on the result you wish to achieve and find someone to hold you accountable.
4. Take the 30-Day Exercise Challenge and never throw in the towel.

"You don't have to be fit and healthy to start
but you do have to start to be fit and healthy."
—Jim Kirwan

CHAPTER 21

ANYONE CAN RUN

My favorite form of exercise is running so I couldn't write this book about exercise without including a chapter about running. I believe that anyone can run if they want to, with very few exceptions. When you were a child, you first learned to walk and then running was the next step. From that point on, you probably spent much of your childhood running around without even thinking about it.

They say you never forget how to ride a bike, which I believe is true but you need a bike. Assuming you are physically able, there is nothing to stop you from running again. It all depends on your attitude; if you are positive and believe that you can, then you can. Whatever you do, do not say you are too old or too heavy to run. *You are not* and there are many, many examples which prove the point; I am sure you can think of a few.

Walking is an enjoyable pastime and I encourage everyone to get out and walk; it is so much better than doing nothing. However, unless you are walking fast (over four miles an hour), you are only exercising at a moderate level and this is really not enough if you want to improve your overall health, increase your life expectancy and with it, your general quality of life. People sometimes ask me what I am training for when they see me running—as if running is only for people doing races. Given the opportunity, I like to say that I am running for my life!

The *2008 Physical Activity Guidelines for Americans* clearly demonstrates that walking at a moderate intensity is just a starting point and that more vigorous exercise is required for increasing life expectancy and quality of life.

Reasons for Running

While walking is good for you, running is even better because of the increased intensity of your exercise. In Chapter 7 we discussed how to make exercise a high priority in your life and I described the many benefits of exercise, but let's take a moment to reconsider just a few of the highlights. Regular physical activity, and especially running, lowers the risks associated with many diseases and conditions including the following:

- Alzheimer's and other dementias
- Anxiety attacks and depression
- High blood pressure
- Cancers, including breast, colon, ovarian, pancreatic, prostate and stomach
- Heart disease
- Osteoporosis
- Sleep apnea and other sleep disorders
- Stroke
- Type 2 diabetes and obesity

While the health benefits alone should persuade you, there are many other reasons why you should consider running. Here are just ten of them that should help motivate you:

10 Great Reasons You Will Love Running

1. You always feel better after running.
2. It's so easy to do; easier than riding a bike.
3. You will lose weight faster than just walking.
4. You can have fun at a relatively low cost.
5. It is great for family relationships.
6. You can make great friends from running and enhance your social life.
7. It is great for taking "time-out" to think, to reflect and to be creative.
8. Running gives you more energy and vitality.
9. You can run outdoors and enjoy the environment.
10. You can run on vacation and explore new places.

Over the years, I have heard many reasons why people think they cannot exercise and all of them apply to running. You can find details about these obstacles to running, and exercise in general, in Chapter 6.

I often hear older folks say, "I can't run because it is too hard for someone of my age" or an overweight person say, "I can't run because it is too hard for someone as heavy as I am". They think that running is for "younger" and "slimmer" people and not suited to folks who are older, overweight or out of shape. It is true that running can be hard, especially at the start, but I believe most people start running in a way which makes it more difficult and less enjoyable than it should be. This leads to a self-fulfilling prophecy that running is too hard, they can't do it, they are too old, too heavy, etc.

So what do most people do wrong when they start running?

In my experience over forty years of running, the single biggest reason people feel it is too hard is because they start out too fast. They move from walking to running but the increase in intensity is too great and they end up having to stop shortly after they start running. This situation is then repeated over and over. While some do persevere and come out of this process as runners, unfortunately far too many fall by the wayside and stop. They understandably feel that running is just too hard, too uncomfortable and that they are just not cut out to run. Consequently, they throw in the towel and quit, often with a very negative attitude towards running and justifiably so, based on their experience.

Most walk-to-run training programs, to one extent or another, fall into the same trap, although with a good coach managing the process and holding you accountable, you have a much better chance of success.

So what is going on here?

Walking

When people are walking, they typically walk somewhere between two and four miles an hour. Put another way, that is a pace of between fifteen and thirty minutes per mile. If you have been walking for a while, you should find thirty-minute miles, maybe even twenty-minute miles, very comfortable. Your breathing will be good, your heart rate will be very comfortable and you will be sweating a little.

You should be able to keep this up for at least thirty minutes to an hour, depending on how long you have been doing it. Table 1 below compares the walking intensity levels from very easy, for folks who are getting back into exercise, to speed walking for more advanced folks. It records speed, distance and per-mile pace, based on a constant time of forty minutes.

TABLE 1

Walking Intensity	Very Easy	Easy	Moderate	Fast	Speed*
Speed (Miles Per Hour)	2.0	2.5	3.5	4.0	5
Mile Pace (Minutes)	30	24	17	15	12
Constant Time (Minutes)	40	40	40	40	40
Distance (Miles)	1.33	1.66	2.33	2.66	3.33

* Speed walking is fast but it does not refer to race walking,
which is faster than most runners.

To help you easily follow the math, the "Moderate Walk" example is set out for you here:

Moderate Walk		
Speed	Given	3.5 MPH
Pace	60 Mins. ÷ 3.5 MPH	17 Mins. Per Mile
Time	Given	40 Mins.
Distance	40 Mins. X 3.5 MPH ÷ 60	2.33 Miles

Your speed is given at 3.5 miles per hour. You calculate your pace in minutes per mile by dividing sixty minutes by 3.5, which gives you a pace of circa seventeen minutes per mile. Your time is forty minutes and this is also given and you calculate your distance by multiplying your time by your speed. Put another way, multiply your speed by two-thirds of an hour.

Running

When people run, they usually run at a pace which is much faster than walking. World-class athletes broke the four-minute mile barrier long ago but the average guy or gal is more likely to be in the seven to fifteen-minutes per mile range. If you start out by trying to run at, say, twelve-minute mile pace, it will feel very uncomfortable if you are used to walking at a relatively slow pace between seventeen and twenty-four-minutes per mile.

The faster you try to run, the more uncomfortable it will be as you move from aerobic exercise into what is called anaerobic territory and this pace will quickly force you to stop because you are not used to this level of intensity.

Table 2 below compares the "Moderate Walking" intensity level from the previous Table 1 with three different levels of running: Slow, Moderate and Fast.

TABLE 2

Intensity	Moderate Walk	Slow Run	Moderate Run	Fast Run
Speed (Miles Per Hour)	3.5	4.0	6.0	8.0
Mile Pace (Minutes)	17:00	15:00	10:00	7:30
Constant Time (Minutes)	40	40	40	40
Distance (Miles)	2.33	2.66	4.0	5.33

Again, to help you follow the math above, the "Slow Run" example is worked out for you here:

Slow Run		
Speed	This is given	4.0 MPH
Pace	60 Mins. ÷ 4 MPH	15 Minutes Per Mile
Time	This is given	40 Minutes
Distance	40 Mins. X 4 MPH ÷ 60	2.67 Miles

Your speed is given at four miles per hour. You calculate your pace in minutes per mile by dividing sixty minutes by four, which gives you a pace of fifteen minutes per mile. Your time at forty minutes is also given and you calculate your distance by multiplying your time by your speed. Put another way, multiply your speed by two-thirds of an hour.

There is no rule which says you have to run faster than you walk!

Did you notice that all the information for the slow run in Table 2 is the same as the fast walk in Table 1? Please check them and you will see that they are identical! What would happen if you start running at a pace that is comfortable enough for you to keep going without having to stop because you are out of breath or because it is too hard?

What would happen if you start to run at your current walking pace?

Table 3 below shows exactly the same speed, pace, time and distance for a "Moderate Walk" and a new running level which we will simply call "Start Running".

Table 3

Intensity	Moderate Walk	Start Running
Speed (Miles Per Hour)	3.5	3.5
Mile Pace (Minutes)	17	17
Time (Minutes)	40	40
Distance (Miles)	2.33	2.33

How do you go from a moderate walk to a slow run without changing your pace?

It seems like a fairly straightforward question but it is much harder to do than you think. Most people will immediately go faster when they start running. It is very hard to find the correct pace, especially when you are not used to running.

There is another requirement before you can comfortably start running. You have to be able to walk before you can run. A bit like an airplane, you need to be traveling fast enough to 'take off' and start running. You must be able to walk at the "Moderate Walk" speed from Table 3 above of 3.5 miles per hour, which is a pace of seventeen minutes per mile. You should be able to do this for at least thirty minutes, which means you can cover a distance of close to two miles in that time.

Once you can walk fast enough, you are ready to start running. So how do you progress to running without changing from your moderate walking pace?

My Unique Approach—Anyone Can Run in 5 Easy Steps

To answer this simple question, I have produced what I believe is a unique but very easy approach, which I call "Anyone Can Run in 5 Easy Steps". Assuming you can walk at a moderate speed of three and a half miles per hour for thirty minutes there is only one last requirement before you can start running.

You must have a partner who can do this with you!

It doesn't really matter who it is, though the ideal partner is someone at the same level as you are, so you can advance through the process together. It could be a more experienced runner but they must understand and be supportive of the process. If you cannot find a partner, you could use a GPS watch to monitor your speed but this is tricky, so I would prefer if you could find a partner.

Step 1: Warm Up, Walking With Your Partner

Warm up by slowly walking together for five minutes at a slow pace and then gradually build your speed up to three and a half miles per hour, which is a little over a seventeen-minute-mile pace. Hold your speed at this level for another five minutes.

Step 2: You Start Running

While your partner continues to walk at the same speed of three and a half miles per hour, you start running. You must stay slightly behind your partner to ensure that it is your partner and not you who controls the pace. This is the critical ingredient which you must follow. If you do, you will be able to run, perhaps very slowly, but still running nonetheless.

Step 3: You Run For 20 Minutes

Your partner continues to walk slightly ahead of you and remains in control of the pace. You continue to run at this seventeen-minute-mile pace for as long as you can but for *no more than* twenty minutes. You may be able to keep running for the full twenty minutes, which means you will have run a little over a mile. If you can only do ten minutes or even five, that is fine. This is already a lot more than you have done before. ***Do not be tempted to increase your speed***; you will have plenty of opportunities to do that later!

Step 4: Your Partner Starts Running

Now swap roles with your partner and repeat step three. They switch from walking to running for up to twenty minutes while you go back to walking again at the same speed. You are now in control of the pace with your partner running slightly behind you.

One thing to remember here is that if your partner is at the same fitness level as you are, they may find the run a little more challenging because they have already walked for some thirty minutes. If this happens, they may have to stop a little earlier and you should simply swap places the next day until you feel confident that you can both run together without going too fast.

Step 5: Cool Down Together

Cool down by walking together, gradually slowing down for ten minutes.

This five-step process does not have to be precise; you should use your watch to time each part but do not worry about your speed at this point. All that matters is that you and your partner each try to run for up to twenty minutes.

Congratulations—you are now a runner and it only took you thirty minutes!

If you would like to learn more about running, I have written an e-book, called *Anyone Can Run* and I have developed a comprehensive eighteen-week training program built around this unique approach. To learn more go to:

www.GetAmericaMoving.com/Anyone-Can-Run.

My unique approach promises to get you up and running for up to twenty minutes in one thirty-minute session, assuming you are already fit enough to start. If you have been inactive but would like to get started you can reach that required level of fitness through a combination of moderate walking and some strength and stretching exercises. Details are set out in *Anyone Can Run*.

Once you get started, I know you will enjoy your running and in anticipation of your success, you can look forward to a long, high quality and healthy life where running is an important part of your new lifestyle.

✗ Your "To Do" List

1. Open your mind and do not say you are too old or too heavy to run.
2. Make sure you can walk for thirty minutes at a moderate pace before you try running.
3. Follow my unique approach to running—Anyone Can Run in 5 Easy Steps.

"Running is the greatest metaphor for life,
because you get out of it what you put into it."
—Oprah Winfrey

RESOURCES

Get America Moving Resources:

Website: www.GetAmericaMoving.com

Blog: www.GetAmericaMoving.com/blog

Facebook: www.Facebook.com/GetAmericaMoving.comWithJimKirwan

Youtube: www.Youtube.com/user/GetAmericaMoving1

Twitter: www.Twitter.com/GetAmericaMovin

Fitness Programs:

30 Day Exercise Challenge (Free Program)

This FREE Challenge is a great way to get started and you can get immediate access to it at **www.GetAmericaMoving.com/challenge**.

5X Fitness Transformation (5XFT)

This is a comprehensive fitness program based on my Exercise BASICS Formula and it comes in a range of options including:

- Starter Package - includes Levels 1 and 2 over 18 weeks
- Complete Package - includes all 5 Levels over 52 weeks

You can get details as **www.GetAmericaMoving.com/5XFT**

Anyone Can Run

This is a comprehensive eighteen-week training program built around my unique approach to start running. To learn more go to **www.GetAmericaMoving. com/Anyone-Can-Run**

Coaching Programs:

5X Lifestyle Mission

You can find out more about my signature coaching program, called 5XLM for short at:

www.GetAmericaMoving.com/5XLM

Other Products:

Exercise BASICS Formula

This is a series of four videos which answers two very important questions:

1. How long should you spend exercising?
2. What type of exercise should you do?

You can find them at **www.GetAmericaMoving.com/basics/.**

Other Resources:

The following include several resources that I have found very helpful in my own personal research, as well as the research I conducted for this book. I would highly recommend that you add at least some of these resources to your "must read" list!

1. *The Blood Sugar Solution: The UltraHealthy Program for Losing Weight, Preventing Disease and Feeling Great Now!* By Mark Hyman, M.D. (2012). New York, NY. Little, Brown and Co.
2. *Eat to Live: The Amazing Nutrient-Rich Program for Fast and Sustained Weight Loss* by Joel Fuhrman, M.D. (2011). New York, NY. Little, Brown and Co.
3. *The End of Dieting: How to Live for Life* by Joel Fuhrman, M.D. (2014). New York, NY. Harper Collins Publishing.

4. *Food is Better Medicine than Drugs: Your Prescription for Drug-Free Health* by Patrick Holford & Jerome Burne. (2006). London. Hachette Digital.

5. *The Great Cholesterol Myth: Why Lowering Your Cholesterol Won't Prevent Heart Disease—and the Statin-Free Plan that Will* by Jonny Bowden, PhD, C.N.S. & Stephen Sinatra, M.D., F.A.C.C. (2012). Beverly, MA. Fair Winds Press.

6. *Performance-Driven Thinking: A Challenging Journey that will Encourage You to Embrace the Greatest Performance of Your Life* by David L. Hancock and Bobby Kipper. (2014). New York, NY. Morgan James Publishing

7. *Running and Being: The Total Experience* by Dr. George Sheehan. (1978). New York, NY. Rodale Inc.

8. *Use Your Brain to Change Your Age: Secrets to Look, Feel, and Think Younger Every Day* by Daniel G. Amen, M.D. (2012). New York, NY. Three Rivers Press.

9. *Younger Next Year: Live Strong, Fit and Sexy—Until You're 80 and Beyond* by Chris Crowley & Henry S. Lodge, M.D. (2005). New York, NY. Workman Publishing Co.

INDEX

5X Fitness Transformation (5XFT), 50, 107, 170, 235

30 Day Exercise Challenge, 222-223, 235

A

Aerobic Exercise (See also Cardio), 31-32, 35, 53, 64, 86-87, 91-98, 103-113, 143, 146, 154, 167, 201, 203, 222, 228

Active Life Expectancy, 37-38

Aging, 3-4, 41-43, 53, 57, 60, 63, 65, 96, 121, 191, 198-199, 203

Alzheimer's, 3, 10-12, 51, 63, 65, 130-131, 185, 188, 190, 193, 197, 199-202, 225

Anaerobic Exercise, 228

Anyone Can Run, 125, 170, 184, 224-233, 236

Aqua Jogging, 55

Arthritis(See also Osteoarthritis), 55-56, 60, 63-64, 225

B

Baseline (See also Unplanned Exercise), 26, 29, 82, 87-93, 103, 105, 142, 214

BASICS, 73-74, 87, 107, 235-236

Benefits of Exercise, 3, 5, 11-12, 16-17, 19-23, 30, 54, 56-61, 63-73, 79-80, 89, 91, 96, 102, 108, 194, 201, 219, 225

Biggest Loser, 7, 34, 54, 59, 120-121, 126, 128, 168, 186, 221

Biking (See also Cycling), 6, 34, 55, 68, 70, 75-76, 81, 84, 86, 91, 93-94, 98-101, 105, 136, 146, 167

Blood Glucose, 10, 21, 189

Blood Pressure, 21, 64, 131, 142, 200, 225

Blood Sugar, 10, 131, 142, 189, 193, 208, 236

Body Mass Index (BMI), 9, 22-23, 62, 135, 140, 145, 186

Body Weight, 23, 62, 66, 76, 84, 87, 89, 94, 135, 140-141, 186,

188-189, 191, 196, 199, 208, 211-215

Brain, 11, 64-65, 87, 183, 186, 191-193, 195-204, 213, 215, 237

Breathing, 74, 144-145, 191-192, 194, 227

C

Calories, 32-33, 66, 84, 89, 96, 193, 196, 201, 208, 210-214

Cancer, 10, 21, 29, 39, 63, 192, 197, 199-200, 225

Cardio (see also Aerobic Exercise), 29-32, 35, 53, 64, 86-87, 91-98, 103-113, 143, 146, 154, 167, 201, 203, 222, 228

Celebrity Apprentice, 188

Centers for Disease Control and Prevention (CDC), 8, 14, 20, 186-187

Chronic Activity Limitations, 37-38, 41

Circuit Training, 86, 94

Cross-Training, 55, 65, 87-88, 92, 94, 99-100, 103, 146

Current Fitness Level, 43, 50, 73, 83, 87, 96, 108, 117, 132, 138-150, 153, 158, 161, 169, 222

Cycling, 6, 34, 55, 68, 70, 75-76, 81, 84, 86, 91, 93-94, 98-101, 105, 136, 146, 167

D

Deep Breathing, 191-192

Dehydration, 200, 213

Dementia, 10, 63, 65, 130-131, 197, 199-200, 225

Diabetes (See also Type 2 Diabetes), 3, 9-12, 29, 51, 63, 66, 131, 135, 185-191, 197, 199-200, 208, 225

Diabesity, 10, 186

Dinosaur Syndrome, 199

Drivers (See also Four Key Drivers), 4, 44-45, 119, 183, 186, 190, 194

E

Exercise B.A.S.I.C.S Formula, 73, 107, 235-236

F

Fartlek, 98

Fitness Program, 50, 63, 73, 93, 96-97, 107, 109-113, 148, 161, 169-170, 222, 232, 235

Flexibility (See also Stretching), 55, 64, 87, 92, 94, 97, 101-103, 106, 143, 163, 232

Four Key Drivers, 4, 44-45, 119, 183, 186, 190, 194

Free Weights, 86,94

G

Get America Moving, 73, 108, 129, 192, 218, 222-223, 232, 236

H

Healthy Charleston Challenge, 7, 54, 120-121, 126, 128, 168

Heart, 10, 25, 29, 31, 39, 51, 54, 56, 63, 65, 74, 87, 126-127, 130-131, 135, 171, 186-188, 191-203, 213, 225, 227, 237

Heart Disease, 10, 29, 39, 51, 56, 63, 65, 130-131, 135, 186-188, 191, 193, 199-200, 225, 237

Heredity, 38-39

High Blood Pressure, 21, 64, 142, 200, 225

Higher intensity (See also Intensity), 16, 21, 32-33, 40, 49, 64-67, 71, 73-81, 84, 87-88, 91-93, 96-100, 103-106, 109-113, 146, 153, 192, 203, 225-230

HIIT (High Intensity Interval Training), 92, 97-98

HR Management; 155, 242

Hydration, 202-203, 213

I

Inactivity Epidemic, 3-4, 11-13, 19, 21, 24-35, 41, 67, 185, 205, 242

Injury, 41, 54-55, 73, 92, 94, 96-97, 99, 102, 121, 126, 130, 135, 157, 178

Insulin Resistance, 10, 188-189, 199

Institute for Integrative Nutrition, 205

Intensity, 16, 21, 32-33, 40, 49, 64-67, 71, 73-81, 84, 87-88, 91-93, 96-100, 103-106, 109-113, 146, 153, 192, 203, 225-230

Intervals, 97-98

J

Jogging, 55, 74-75, 86, 91, 105, 178

K

Knowledge, 44-46, 119, 181, 183-193

L

Life Expectancy, 4, 13, 19, 21-23, 35-43, 57, 96, 117, 120-121, 131, 135, 189, 198, 217, 223, 225, 242

Lifestyle Mission (See also Mission), 129-140, 149, 152, 159, 166, 170, 174, 176, 179, 191, 198, 203, 214, 236

M

Marathon, 6, 70, 100, 126-127, 136, 153, 157, 165, 177-178, 242

Medical Clearance, xviii, 140

MET (Metabolic Equivalent Task), 75-85, 105-106, 109-113, 146

Metabolism, 32, 66, 84, 87, 96, 212, 214-215

Mild Cognitive Impairment (MCI), 196, 199-200

Mission (See also Lifestyle Mission),129-140, 149, 152, 159,

166, 170, 174, 176, 179, 191, 198, 203, 214, 236

Muscle Mass, 12, 41, 66, 95-96

Muscle Strengthening (See also Strength), 12, 16-17, 32, 40, 55, 64, 66, 77-79, 86-87, 92-96, 99, 102-103, 105-106, 109-113, 128, 143, 146, 163, 194, 201, 203, 232

N

Nutrition, 8, 29, 44-46, 90, 119, 121, 131, 136-137, 150, 155, 183-185, 190-191, 203, 205-216

O

Obese (Obesity), 3, 7, 8-12, 21-23, 30, 39, 62, 130-131, 140-142, 185-188, 191, 199-200, 208-209, 225

Osteoarthritis, 55-56, 60, 63-64, 225

Overweight, 7-9, 12, 21-23, 39, 53, 58, 62, 66, 91, 131, 140-141, 186-187, 191, 199, 209, 214, 221, 226

P

Physical Activity Guidelines, 15-22, 30, 72-79, 109, 225

Planned Exercise, 26-27, 35, 53, 70, 88, 90-92, 104, 142

Pre Diabetes, 10-11, 66, 131, 188-191, 197-200, 208, 225

Projects, 123, 127-128,131-132, 136-138, 150-155, 165, 170, 172, 175, 178

Q

Quality of Life, 3, 19, 35-40, 43-45, 49, 57, 59, 69, 87, 91, 96, 107, 117, 119-121, 130-135, 177, 184, 194, 198-199, 211, 214, 217, 223-225, 232, 242

R

R.E.C.I.P.E. 117, 122-123, 132-133, 138, 153

Road Race, 98, 128, 134, 136, 150, 153-154, 158-159, 161-162, 166, 170, 172-177, 192

Rugby, 8, 26-28, 86, 90, 178

Running, 6, 26, 28, 34, 56, 58, 65, 68-70, 75-81, 86-87, 91, 93-95, 98-101, 105, 124-128, 136,143, 146-147, 150, 153, 156, 163, 165, 167, 169, 178-179, 184, 195, 201, 218, 224-233, 236-237, 241-242

S

Sarcopenia, 64, 66, 95-96

Sitting the New Smoking, 29, 90, 142

Skiing, 68, 70, 86, 91, 93-94, 98,100,105, 167

Sleep, 29, 54, 63, 65, 88-89,130, 142, 145, 166, 191-192, 194, 197, 199-200, 202-203, 225

Slippery Slope, 41-44
Smart Goals, 137, 159, 161, 167
Speed Work, 97-98
Spinning, 53, 55, 169
Strength, 12, 16-17, 32, 40, 55, 64,
    66, 77-79, 86-87, 92-96, 99,
    102-103, 105-106, 109-113, 128,
    143, 146, 163, 194, 201, 203,
    232
Stress, 63, 65, 69, 130, 145, 200,
    202, 215
Stretching (see also Flexibility), 55,
    64, 87, 92, 94, 97, 101-103, 106,
    143, 163, 232
Stroke, 10, 51, 63, 188, 191, 197,
    199-200, 225
Supplements, 194, 202
Swimming, 6, 26, 28, 34, 55, 68, 70,
    86-87, 91, 93-94, 98-100, 105,
    136, 143, 146, 167, 169, 171,
    209, 241

T
Tempo, 98
The Biggest Loser (See also Biggest
    Loser), 7, 34, 54, 59, 120-121,
    126, 128, 168, 186, 221
Training Program, 32, 50, 55, 96-97,
    127-128, 161-162, 164, 169-170,
    172, 176, 227, 232, 236, 242
Triathlon, 6, 27, 56, 70, 87, 100-101,
    126, 136, 153, 157, 165, 171,
    175, 241-242

Type 2 Diabetes, 3, 9-12, 29, 51, 63,
    66, 131, 135, 185-191, 197, 199-
    200, 208, 225
Type 3 Diabetes, 10
TrySports, 6, 120, 129-130, 241-242

U
Unplanned Exercise (See also
    Baseline), 26, 29, 82, 87-93, 103,
    105, 142, 214

V
Visceral Fat, 10, 189
Vitamin D, 192

W
Waist to Height Ratio, 140-141, 145
Waist to Hips Ratio, 141-142, 145
Walking, 6, 58, 70, 75-81, 86, 88-91,
    94, 99, 101, 105, 109-110, 127-
    128, 136, 143-147, 150, 153,
    157, 163, 165, 169, 218, 222,
    224-232, 241
Water, 40, 68, 70, 89, 163, 196, 200-
    203, 206, 213-214, 216
Whole Foods, 202, 206, 212, 215-
    216
World Health Organization, 20-22,
    72

X
X Factor, 44-45, 117, 119-133
X Man, 120-121

ABOUT THE AUTHOR

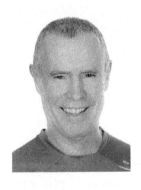

Jim Kirwan is the founder and former CEO of TrySports and the creator of Get America Moving. He came to the United States from Ireland in 2003 to set up TrySports, a specialty retail business focused on the aerobic activities of walking, running, swimming, cycling, fitness and triathlon. The first store opened its doors in 2004 in Mount Pleasant, South Carolina and quickly demonstrated that it was no ordinary retail store. Led by the founder, TrySports got actively involved in the health and fitness of the local community and quickly won a reputation for providing great customer service and for inspiring thousands to get fit and live a healthy life.

After opening a second store in 2007 in Charlotte, North Carolina, TrySports' two stores were voted the second and third best specialty running stores in the nation the following year by the readers of *Runner's World*, one of the leading running magazines in the world. Two further store openings in 2008 led to TrySports becoming an INC 5000 "fastest growing company" for 3 years in a row from 2009 to 2011.

244 | THE EXERCISE FACTOR

As time passed, Jim became so concerned about the health problems facing America that with TrySports poised for continued growth, he decided to step down as CEO at the end of 2012 and he is now on a mission to Get America Moving. He coined the phrase the "Inactivity Epidemic" because the vast majority of Americans don't exercise enough and he worries that in a few short years we will look back and wonder, a bit like smoking, how we failed to connect the dots about our inactivity. While there are no guarantees in life, he believes you can significantly influence your life expectancy and the quality of your life by the actions you take now.

At the start of 2014 he created Get America Moving and in April 2014 he launched his first product, "5X Fitness Transformation", a comprehensive, fifty-two week exercise program that is broken down into five progressive Levels and is designed for you regardless of your age, weight or current fitness level. Besides writing *The eXercise Factor*, he is working on another book as well as his first coaching program.

Jim Kirwan is so passionate about Get America Moving, that he has recently appeared on television many times, including Fox 5 News in Las Vegas, NBC in Tampa & Palm Springs, Kron 4 in San Francisco, ABC in Albuquerque (which included a 5 part series) and, of course, ABC News 4 in Charleston, his home town!

Before he came to America he worked for eighteen years with Ireland's leading bank, the Bank of Ireland, in a wide range of personnel management roles. He left the bank in 1990 to set up his first business, a successful personnel management consultancy, based in Dublin, providing a range of services including recruitment and selection, performance management, training and development and remuneration.

Jim Kirwan went to Belvedere College in Dublin, one of Ireland's leading secondary schools famous for another James, the author James Joyce. He graduated from University College Dublin with a B. Comm (Honors) in 1977. He is a fellow of the Chartered Institute of Personnel and Development (UK and Ireland). He has completed four marathons, many triathlons and has many years' experience coaching running, cross-country, track and field and triathlon.

Printed in the USA
CPSIA information can be obtained
at www.ICGtesting.com
JSHW022219140824
68134JS00018B/1150